T0226897

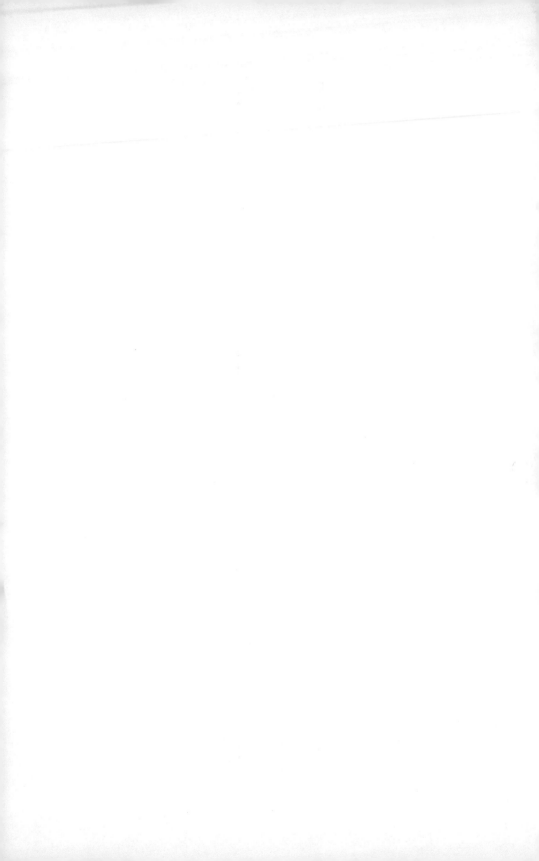

Orthopedic Nursing

Editor

TANDY GABBERT

NURSING CLINICS OF NORTH AMERICA

www.nursing.theclinics.com

Consulting Editor
STEPHEN D. KRAU

June 2020 • Volume 55 • Number 2

ELSEVIER

1600 John F. Kennedy Boulevard • Suite 1800 • Philadelphia, Pennsylvania, 19103-2899

http://www.theclinics.com

NURSING CLINICS OF NORTH AMERICA Volume 55, Number 2
June 2020 ISSN 0029-6465, ISBN-13: 978-0-323-69563-3

Editor: Kerry Holland
Developmental Editor: Casey Potter

Nursing Clinics of North America (ISSN 0029-6465) is published quarterly by Elsevier Inc., 360 Park Avenue South, New York, NY 10010-1710. Months of issue are March, June, September, and December. Periodicals postage paid at New York, NY and additional mailing offices. Subscription price per year is, $163.00 (US individuals), $518.00 (US institutions), $275.00 (international individuals), $631.00 (international institutions), $231.00 (Canadian individuals), $631.00 (Canadian institutions), $100.00 (US and Canadian students), and $135.00 (international students). To receive student/resident rate, orders must be accompanied by name of affiliated institution, date of term, and the signature of program/residency coordinator on institution letterhead. Orders will be billed at individual rate until proof of status is received. Foreign air speed delivery is included in all *Clinics* subscription prices. All prices are subject to change without notice. **POSTMASTER:** Send address changes to *Nursing Clinics*, Elsevier Health Sciences Division, Subscription Customer Service, 3251 Riverport Lane, Maryland Heights, MO 63043. **Customer Service: Telephone: 1-800-654-2452** (U.S. and Canada); **1-314-447-8871 (outside U.S. and Canada). Fax: 1-314-447-8029. E-mail: journalscustomerservice-usa@ elsevier.com** (for print support) and **journalsonlinesupport-usa@elsevier.com** (for online support).

Nursing Clinics of North America is covered in *EMBASE/Excerpta Medica, MEDLINE/PubMed (Index Medicus), Social Sciences Citation Index, Current Contents, ASCA, Cumulative Index to Nursing, RNdex Top 100,* and Allied Health Literature and International Nursing Index (INI).

Contributors

CONSULTING EDITOR

STEPHEN D. KRAU, PhD, RN, CNE
Associate Professor (Ret), Vanderbilt University School of Nursing, Nashville, Tennessee

EDITOR

TANDY GABBERT, MSN, RN, ONC
Director of Education, National Association of Orthopaedic Nurses, Chicago, Illinois

AUTHORS

HEATHER C. BARNES, DNP, APRN, CPNP, ONC
Certified Pediatric Nurse Practitioner, Department of Orthopaedic Surgery and Musculoskeletal Science, Section of Sports Medicine, Children's Mercy Kansas City, Kansas City, Missouri

DEBRA BYRD, BSN, RN, ONC
Orthopedic Clinical Care Coordinator, Specialty Service Lines, AdventHealth, Celebration, Florida

CAROLYN CRANE CUTILLI, PhD, RN-BC
Patient Education Specialist, Hospital of the University of Pennsylvania, Philadelphia, Pennsylvania; Adjunct Nursing Professor, American International College, Springfield, Massachusetts

KARI L. BAERWALD ERICKSON, BAN, RN, ONC
RN Program Specialist, Orthopedics, Sanford Medical Center Fargo, Fargo, North Dakota

KIMBERLY K. HAYNES, RN, DNP, MS, ACNS-BC, ONC, APRN
Clinical Nurse Specialist, The University of Kansas Hospital Sarcoma Center, Overland Park, Kansas

PATRICIA IYER, MSN, RN, LNCC
Past National President, American Association of Legal Nurse Consultants, Chicago, Illinois; President, The Pat Iyer Group, Fort Myers, Florida

BARBARA J. LEVIN, BSN, RN, ONC, CMSRN, LNCC
Clinical Scholar Orthopaedic Trauma Unit, Massachusetts General Hospital, Chair, Massachusetts Board of Registration in Nursing, Boston, Massachusetts; Past National President, American Association of Legal Nurse Consultants, Past National Director, National Association of Orthopedic Nurses, Chicago, Illinois

SALLY H. PEARSON, DNP, FNP, ONC
Associate Professor, Mississippi University for Women, Columbus, Mississippi

DOROTHY PIETROWSKI, MSN, ACNP, ONP-C
Orthopaedic Nurse Practitioner, Department of Orthopaedic Surgery and Rehabilitative Services, University of Chicago, Chicago, Illinois

HOWARD G. ROSENTHAL, MD, FACS
Medical Director, Sarcoma Center, The University of Kansas Hospital Sarcoma Center, Overland Park, Kansas

DEBRA L. SIETSEMA, MSN, PhD
Director, Bone Health Clinical Operations, The CORE Institute, Director, Grants and Education, MORE Foundation, Phoenix, Arizona

ADAM STEPHAN, MSN, RN
Assistant Vice President, Orthopedic Service Line, HCA – Gulf Coast Division, National Association of Orthopaedic Nursing, Chicago, Illinois

RACHEL TORANI, MSN, MBA, BSN, RN
Regional Director of the Orthopedic Institute, AdventHealth, Orlando, Florida

ANGELA C. VANDERPOOL, MSN, APRN, CPNP, ONC
Certified Pediatric Nurse Practitioner, Department of Orthopaedic Surgery and Musculoskeletal Science, Section of Sports Medicine, Children's Mercy Kansas City, Kansas City, Missouri

MICHAEL E. ZYCHOWICZ, DNP, ANP, ONP, FAAN, FAANP
Professor of Nursing Lead Faculty, Orthopedic NP Specialty, Duke University School of Nursing, Durham, North Carolina

Contents

> Wellness care should start when the diagnosis of osteoarthritis becomes evident. Guidelines from the American Academy of Orthopaedic Surgeons and the American College of Rheumatology are the basis of the treatment modalities. Providing patients with intentional strategies to prepare them for possible joint replacement surgery is key to prevent postoperative complications and give them the best opportunity for an optimal outcome after surgical intervention. The Clinical Guidelines for Nonsurgical Management of Osteoarthritis algorithm helps providers with the implementation of these strategies. The primary focus is to help providers be proactive instead of reactive in osteoarthritis care.

> Hip fractures that occur in the elderly population continue to be a growing problem in communities. In this particular population, people 65 years and older, patients often have multiple comorbidities. These comorbidities cause challenges for a patient's optimization preoperatively and throughout the continuum of care. Although unplanned and traumatic, hip fracture patients can benefit from care organized in a comprehensive and standardized way. Having a hip fracture program that is driven by a multidisciplinary team approach has proved to decrease length of stay and promote positive outcomes for patients.

> Nurse practitioners (NPs) play an increasingly greater role in the delivery of orthopedic patient care. NPs practice in a wide variety of orthopedic settings having a significant positive impact on orthopedic care delivery. Few formal educational outlets exist for training NPs for orthopedic care. Many new orthopedic NPs rely on continuing education and an apprenticeship model of learning "on the job" with their surgeon counterparts. This article describes the preparation, role, and impact that today's NPs have on orthopedic care delivery.

Total joint replacement (TJR) is one of the most commonly performed and painful surgeries in the United States. Over the past few decades, regulatory changes increased the use of oral narcotics as a first-line treatment of this population. In the current opioid crisis, new pain management techniques and therapies have emerged. Research of current therapies, their effectiveness, and emerging best practices are discussed. Clear, thoughtful, and thorough education is an essential next step for closing the gap of the pain experience. Specifically, education of the frontline nurses, patients, and their caregivers on pain reduction techniques is essential.

Over the past several decades there has been a dramatic change in the landscape of youth sports. This article provides an overview of sport-related injuries in the child and adolescent populations, looking at changes over the past 10 to 15 years. A closer look at frequently seen injuries, including assessment, diagnosis, and management in osteochondritis dissecans, sprains, fractures, anterior cruciate ligament, and meniscus tears, is provided. Current protocols and screening tools for this population are discussed, including pre-participation screening. The nursing implications in the clinical and community setting are identified, with ways to incorporate this information into practice.

The treatment of malignant bone tumors, also called bone sarcomas, has changed dramatically over the past 50 years owing to the advances in chemotherapy, immunotherapy, targeted therapy, radiation, prosthetic technology, and surgical advances. There are 3 main primary bone cancers: osteosarcoma, Ewing's sarcoma (or Ewing's family of sarcoma), and chondrosarcoma. Before advances in limb preservation techniques and before the development of prosthetic replacement, the treatment for a malignant bone tumor of the extremity was amputation. This article discusses the progression of surgical treatment of malignant bone cancers.

The patient education process has 4 equal components to be addressed by the nurse: assessment, planning, implement, and evaluation. Excellent patient education is an "art" and "science" using nuances and evidence-based strategies to effectively educate. The assessment and evaluation components often use nuanced approaches (motivational interviewing, teach back) to engage the patient/caregiver respectfully, whereas planning and implementation rely more on evidence-based strategies such as the Patient Education Assessment of Materials. Nurses should provide education that is simple, patient centered, and multimodal to meet the health literacy needs of patients/caregivers.

NURSING CLINICS OF NORTH AMERICA

SERIES OF RELATED INTEREST

Critical Care Nursing Clinics of North America
https://www.ccnursing.theclinics.com/

THE CLINICS ARE AVAILABLE ONLINE!
Access your subscription at:
www.theclinics.com

Foreword

Osteoporosis: A Prototype for Orthopedic Degenerative Processes

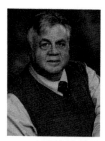

Stephen D. Krau, PhD, RN, CNE
Consulting Editor

As our population ages, there are many health care issues that emerge. It is well known that the elderly are more prone to polypharmacy and that prescribed drug-related issues among the US population have been more catastrophic for the elderly, with the exception perhaps of the matters associated with the opioid epidemic. More than half of the individuals who are over the age of 50 have some semblance of bone compromise, be it overall bone health, osteoporosis, or osteopenia. As the prevalence of these issues continues to rise, it is anticipated that fractures related to fragility will increase as the age of the population increases.[1] It follows that the need for treatment expertise, and financial resources will exponentially increase as issues related to bone health increase. Patients who are admitted for other health care diseases often present with comorbidities related to bone health.

Osteoporosis is the most common human bone disease.[2] It is estimated that 54% of persons 50 and over, which constitutes 43.4 million Americans, have low bone density, and about 10.2 million Americans have osteoporosis. It is predicted that approximately 50% of Caucasian women and 20% of men will experience osteoporotic fractures of the hip, wrist, or spine in their lifetime.[2,3] Internationally, the highest annual age-standardized hip fractures (per 100,000 person-years) was as follows: The highest were found in Scandinavia: Denmark (574), Norway (563), and Sweden (539), plus Austria (501). The lowest were found in closer to the equator in countries such as Nigeria (2), South Africa (20), Tunisa (58), and Ecudor (73).[4]

Despite the advances in the diagnosis of osteoporosis, the development of tools to identify risk of fractures, and multiple treatment modalities, research, and policy development, only a minority of men and women who are at risk for fractures actually receive treatment. The mortality subsequent to a hip fracture is significant with a 2.8 to 4.0

Nurs Clin N Am 55 (2020) ix–x
https://doi.org/10.1016/j.cnur.2020.02.013
0029-6465/20/© 2020 Published by Elsevier Inc.

nursing.theclinics.com

Table 1
Collaborative approach to treating osteoporosis

Universal recommendations	1. Regular weight-bearing exercises 2. Physical activity to aid in balance, strength, and posture 3. Patient education related to bone density, fracture risk, weight-bearing activities, spine care, avoidance of heaving lifting, bending, or twisting
Pharmacologic management	1. Calcium and vitamin D 2. Biophosphates 3. Anti-RANKL 4. Selective estrogen receptor modulator 5. Anabolic agents 6. Sclerostin inhibitor

Adapted from Good SC, Wright TF, Lynch C. Osteoporosis screening and treatment: a colloaborative approach. JNP 2020;16(1):60-63.

times greater incidence within the first 3 months after fracture than similarly aged patients without a hip fracture. The reasons for this are plentiful and include issues such as loss of independence, habitation transfer from independent living to nursing homes, and a myriad of mental health sequalae related to loss of autonomy, fear of falling, and a sense of isolation.

Goode and colleagues[1] have recently proposed a collaborative approach to managing osteoporosis and osteopenia. They propose that the greatest impact on these processes occurs when there are health care personnel available and skilled to ameliorate the outcomes associated with fragility fracture outcomes. In addition, they propose a collaborative approach to treating patients with osteoporosis and osteopenia. **Table 1** presents the overall process by which health care providers can improve outcomes for this population.

Osteoporosis and associated fragility fractures are global issues. Screening, diagnosing, and treating osteoporosis are multilayered endeavors. There have been numerous medications, policies, and tools developed in recent years to ameliorate and treat the incidence of osteoporosis.

Stephen D. Krau, PhD, RN, CNE
Vanderbilt University School of Nursing
6809 Highland Park Drive
Nashville, TN 37205, USA

E-mail address:
sdkrau@outlook.com

REFERENCES

1. Goode SC, Wright TF, Lynch C. Osteoporosis screening and treatment: a collaborative approach. J Nurs Pract 2020;16(1):60–3.
2. US Department of Health and Human Services. Bone health and osteoporosis: a report of the Surgeon General. Rockville (MD): US Department of Health and Human Services, Office of the Surgeon General; 2004.
3. Cosman F, de Beur SJ, LeBoff MS, et al. Clinicians guide to prevention and treatment of osteoporosis. Ostoporos Int 2014;25(10):2359–81.
4. Kanis JA, Odén A, McCloskey EV. A systematic review of hip fracture incidence and probability of fracture worldwide. Osteoporos Int 2012;23(9):2239–56.

Preface

A Vital Specialty for the Twenty-First Century

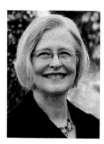

Tandy Gabbert, MSN, RN, ONC
Editor

Caring for patients in their most vulnerable moments is a sacred trust. Providing the highest-quality nursing care based on current evidence is a compelling responsibility. Today's complicated health care landscape mandates a rapid pace of change to accommodate the most up-to-date regulations, evidence, and best practices. Caring for patients with varied musculoskeletal conditions requires a specialized body of knowledge and expertise. Skilled and knowledgeable nurses are empowered to provide excellent care, intervene to prevent injuries and complications, and maintain safety for the staff and for the patient. It is with these thoughts in mind that this issue was developed, offering insight into the diverse variety found in the specialty of Orthopedic Nursing. The authors represent the specialty through their expert roles as nurse practitioners, clinical nurse specialists, direct care providers, faculty, legal nurse consultants, administrators, education consultants, and program specialists. All but one of the authors are members of the National Association of Orthopaedic Nurses, a nurse specialty organization whose mission is to advance the specialty of orthopedic nursing through excellence in research, education, and nursing practice. Find us on the Web at http://www.orthonurse.org.

Orthopedic nursing is a specialty that focuses on musculoskeletal diseases and disorders. The scope of orthopedic conditions is very broad. In this issue, you will find topics related to the role of the advanced practice nurse in orthopedics, spine care innovations, pain management, sports injuries and the adolescent athlete, limb salvage surgery for tumors, legal implications for the orthopedic nurse, tips and "pearls" for patient education, and more.

Across the lifespan, orthopedic conditions intersect readily and often. The articles in this issue carry relevance for nursing practice as well as for personal and family health and wellness. For example:

Nurs Clin N Am 55 (2020) xi–xii
https://doi.org/10.1016/j.cnur.2020.02.012
0029-6465/20/© 2020 Published by Elsevier Inc.

- Osteoarthritis is a leading cause of disability, and its incidence is rising due to increasing obesity and an aging population. The condition and related risk factors are complex and provide a challenge to the managing provider(s). Progress toward adoption of public health prevention interventions is moving slowly.[1] However, proactive wellness care is possible for the patient with this disease.
- Total joint replacement (TJR) is one of the most commonly performed, elective surgical procedures in the United States, and the volume of TJR procedures has risen continuously in recent decades. Over the next 10 years, by 2030, total hip replacement volumes are projected to grow 171%, and total knee replacement is projected to grow by up to 189%, for a projected 635,000 and 1.28 million procedures, respectively.[2] Given this sobering statistic, knowledge about current trends and practices is essential, especially if the patient is a parent or friend.
- Osteoporosis, which literally means porous bone, is a disease in which the density and quality of bone are reduced. As bones become more porous and fragile, the risk of fracture is greatly increased. The loss of bone occurs silently and progressively. Often there are no symptoms until the first fracture occurs. Due to its prevalence worldwide, osteoporosis is considered a worldwide public health concern.[3]
- If you are over the age of 50, especially if you are also a woman, you may be at risk for a fragility fracture. A hip fracture is a serious injury, with complications that can be life-threatening. The risk of hip fracture rises with age and carries serious morbidity. Today's evidence-based protocols for hip fracture care have reduced morbidity significantly.[4,5]

Great thought and research were put into the development of this issue. I commend the authors, experts in their field, for their hard work and dedication to produce this excellent collection of topics. It is truly a pleasure to provide this issue and share "our world."

Orthopedically yours,

Tandy Gabbert, MSN, RN, ONC
4120 West 47th Terrace
Roeland Park, KS 66205, USA

E-mail address:
tandy.gabbert@gmail.com

REFERENCES

1. Johnson VL, Hunter D. The epidemiology of osteoarthritis. Best Pract Rese Clin Rheumatol 2014;28(1):5–15.
2. Sloan M, Sheth N. Projected volume of primary and revision total joint arthroplasty in the United States, 2030-2060. Presented at the Annual Meeting of the American Academy of Orthopaedic Surgeons. New Orleans, LA, March 6, 2018.
3. International Osteoporosis Foundation. Osteoporosis facts and statistics. Available at: https://www.iofbonehealth.org/facts-statistics. Accessed August 1, 2019.
4. Frost SA, Nguyen ND, Black DA, et al. Risk factors for in-hospital post-hip fracture mortality. Bone 2011;49:553.
5. Morrison RS, Siu AL, Schmader KE, et al. Hip fracture in adults: epidemiology and medical management. Available at: https://www.uptodate.com/contents/hip-fracture-in-adults-epidemiology-and-medical-management. Accessed August 1, 2019.

Proactive Wellness Care for Patients with Osteoarthritis

Sally H. Pearson, DNP, FNP, ONC*

KEYWORDS

- Osteoarthritis • Guidelines • Nonsurgical interventions • Modalities • AAOS • ACR

KEY POINTS

- Health care providers need to gain evidence-based knowledge of effective strategies and specific treatment modalities that will assist arthritic patients to improve their overall health.
- Nonsurgical management of osteoarthritis includes exercise, tai chi, weight loss or maintenance, self-management, thermal modalities, and pharmacologic agents. Core strengthening and weight loss may prevent surgery in some cases.
- Preoperative wellness care should begin early and continue in patients with osteoarthritis even after referral to orthopedic surgery. Evaluation for anemia, dental issues, sleep apnea, osteoporosis, and deconditioning should begin when a diagnosis of osteoarthritis is discovered. Attention to these issues can prevent postoperative complications.

INTRODUCTION

"I wish someone had told me." These were the words heard after finishing a doctoral project and telling a friend about the findings. The project was researching whether nurse practitioners (NPs) were discussing proactive therapies with their patients with osteoarthritis (OA), most of whom will eventually have a total knee or hip replacement. Early in the disease process, or even while they are waiting for the disease to progress, was anyone telling them about things they could do to prevent or slow the progression of the disease and get ready for a joint replacement if needed?

Can you relate to an overworked nurse practitioner? My friend was a nurse practitioner in women's health for 25 years. About 3 years before retirement she began to have pain in both hips. She had gained some weight over the years with working long hours and working in a fast-paced clinic. Most of her days consisted of sitting on a rolling stool performing pelvic examinations, then standing to look under the microscope, then back on the stool to complete the conversation with her patient. Repetitive actions daily for more than 20 years began to take their toll. She was eventually diagnosed with OA, resulting in both of her hips being replaced. Complications with 1 surgery delayed her activity level

Mississippi University for Women, Columbus, MS, USA
* Corresponding author. 1100 College Street, Box 910, Columbus, MS 39759.
E-mail address: sallybsa@aol.com

after surgery, and she still walks with a limp 2 years later, and, yes, she has gained more weight with her inactive lifestyle. This stage was when she said, "I wish someone had told me how to get more physically fit and be more prepared for these surgeries. Who knows, I may have made some changes and prevented the progression of this arthritis had I started earlier. I just didn't think about it."

PROBLEM

Researchers have found that, even with a small amount of education on evidence-based guidelines for OA, providers become more assertive. Providers reported more intentional discussions and directions with their patients on how to live with and, it is hoped, prevent the progression of the disease.[1]

Health care providers working in orthopedics have a specialty perspective. However, primary care providers are seeing patients with comorbid conditions, along with arthritis, and may overlook their arthritis until they become more symptomatic. It is not unusual for patients to avoid discussing their sore knees or increasing stiffness until it greatly affects their lifestyles. Nor is it unusual for practitioners to be so involved in acute care or chronic illnesses such as hypertension and diabetes that joint discomfort takes a "back seat" to these more acute issues. There is only so much time in a day and in an office visit. When a problem is mentioned, if nonsteroidal antiinflammatory drugs (NSAIDs) or physical therapy cannot take care of the issue, the patient is usually referred to orthopedics. Once referred, temporary relief can be achieved from intra-articular injections. However, most cases eventually require surgery, with not much in between. The question is, could more be done before surgery?

BURDEN OF DISEASE

In the United States alone, 54.4 million or 1 in 4 adults are affected by arthritis as of 2015 according to the Centers for Disease Control and Prevention (CDC).[2] This number is almost equivalent to the combined 2018 population of California (39.5 million), Mississippi (3 million), Alabama (4.8 million), Louisiana (4.6 million), and Arkansas (3 million).[3] That is a lot of people with arthritis. There are more than 100 different forms of arthritis, with the 2 major forms being OA and rheumatoid arthritis. Out of those two, 27 million Americans have OA.[4] OA leads to many people having increasing pain and physical limitations, which lead to lost time from work and decreased income. OA can be attributed to 25% of all visits to primary care, with half of all NSAID prescriptions being for OA. For every 50 primary care patient visits, 2 are for OA complaints. Most practitioners do not go a day without prescribing NSAIDs.[5]

GUIDELINES

What would have helped my friend? She described at least 3 years of visits with her primary care provider, physical therapist, and several orthopedic surgeons. Even though she is a nurse practitioner, she failed to consider other treatment options for herself. A patient-centered plan with a few goals and problem-solving strategies would have better prepared her for the inevitable total joint arthroplasty. No one helped her "shoot" for the target she had in mind managing her disease. Instead, it managed her.

So how do clinicians help patients hit the target? They need to know where they are aiming; this is where evidence-based guidelines come in. Rheumatologists and orthopedic surgeons manage OA on a daily basis. Who better to advise the primary care providers on this disease management? These organizations specialize in OA care from a medical management perspective with the possible end result of surgical intervention. Primary care providers can benefit from the knowledge and expertise these two specialties provide.

After researching more than 36 different guidelines to treat OA, the search was narrowed to The American Academy of Orthopaedic Surgeons (AAOS) *Treatment of Osteoarthritis of the Knee, Second Edition* (2013),[6] AAOS *Surgical Management of Osteoarthritis of the Knee: Evidence-based Clinical Practice Guidelines* (2015),[7] AAOS *Management of Osteoarthritis of the Hip* (2017),[8] and The *American College of Rheumatology 2012 Recommendations for the Use of Nonpharmacologic and Pharmacologic Therapies in Osteoarthritis of the Hand, Hip, and Knee* (2012).[9] Updated clinical guidelines from AAOS are scheduled to be released in spring 2020 and the American College of Rheumatology (ACR) guidelines are scheduled to be released in 2019.

When looking at guidelines, it is important to understand the guideline language of strong, moderate, limited, consensus grades, and inconclusive. The strength of evidence is based on the number and quality of the studies reviewed. Consensus is an opinion given in the absence of reliable evidence. Inconclusive means there was not enough evidence at that time to have an opinion. Most guidelines are based on recent studies from the last 5 years or the last time the guidelines were updated.[6]

IMPLEMENTING GUIDELINES

There is no room for being a "Lone Ranger" in implementing these guidelines. Even the Lone Ranger had a good horse, Silver, and a companion, Tonto, to achieve the job (**Fig. 1**). You must engage the clinic, including the front desk personnel, medical assistants, and nurses. Teach them to recognize or identify patients at risk, such as those patients with a history of previous trauma, sports-associated injury, repetitive overuse, obesity, positive family history, aging, and complaints of everyday wear and tear on the joint.[4]

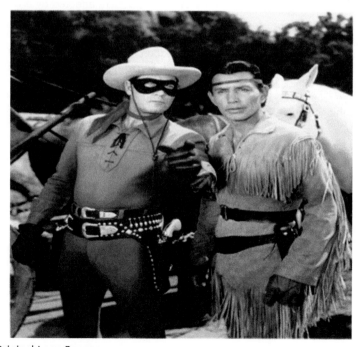

Fig. 1. Original Lone Ranger.

Communicate with the office personnel what your priorities and expectations are but also communicate with your patient. Despite the importance of getting the patient's history, clinicians frequently interrupt the patients before they can fully describe their symptoms.

Beckman and Frankel[10] from 1984 showed that 75% of caregivers interrupt their patients within 18 seconds and an average of 1 concern expressed. When asked, "Is there is anything else you need?" before leaving the room, patients rarely add anything but believe they have been heard. Consider structuring visits to promote communication, and taking time to listen to let patients tell their stories. Include the patients in goal setting and problem-solving strategies. This approach helps patients begin to be engaged in their care. If no goals are set, then they probably will not achieve the target, be it weight loss, decreased pain, increased flexibility, or just slowing the progression of the disease.

Providers must stay up to date. Even the Lone Ranger and Tonto are up to date (**Fig. 2**). Educate your staff, yourself, and your patients. There are areas that help a clinic successfully treat patients with OA. One of the best assets is a competent nurse or medical assistant. Providers should help staff become familiar with evidence-based guidelines and give them the freedom and encouragement to initiate nonpharmacologic management in collaboration with the primary care provider. Encourage office staff to be involved. A strong clinic nurse can make a big difference in patient care. When nurses take the initiative to give patients the tools needed to implement self-care of OA, better outcomes are achieved. Nurses have the prime opportunity to assist these patients as they interact with them in the clinic setting. They can establish a rapport with patients and begin to evaluate their level of disease, and educate the patients on simple but effective ways to enhance their lifestyles.

RESOURCES

There is currently no cure for OA; if efforts are made early to decrease pain while increasing activity and overall wellness, then disease progression may be slowed.[4] Resources are important in the clinic. Use a resource sheet to link the patient to community self-management programs. **Box 1**[11] is an example of a resource list for use with patients in a clinic. Having easy access to facilities and Web sites on 1 resource may increase referrals and encourage clinic personnel involvement. It is easy to create and keeps things simple for patients and office personnel. Providers should engage

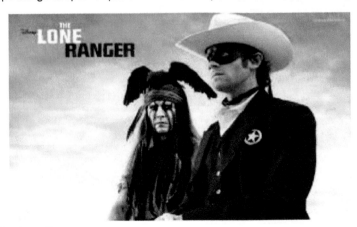

Fig. 2. New Lone Ranger.

their nurses or office personnel to make a handout of local resources for the practice area. If the clinic staff are involved, then they will buy into the process and make it their own. An excellent resource for improving overall management of chronic illnesses in a primary care clinic is the Web site www.improvingchroniccare.org. This site is based on the chronic care model, which helps with system changes to affect care by moving from a reactive style of care to a proactive style. Having a proactive style for chronic illness care can lead to a clinic becoming a community resource. The nurses and clinic staff can build confidence to care more creatively for patients and be empowered to promote community networking. This ability to network and involve local resources adds to the reputation of the clinic and even potentially increases referrals into the clinic with the primary goal of maximizing patient care for the best outcomes.

TREATMENT MODALITIES

Evidence-based guidelines can give direction for intentional care and help medical personnel set goals with patients. An algorithm made from the AAOS and ACR guidelines, Clinical Algorithm for Nonsurgical Management of Osteoarthritis (**Fig. 3**),[1] can serve as a clinical tool.

These guidelines are discussed here, beginning with nonpharmacologic recommendations for exercise, weight control, self-management programs, thermal agents, and tai chi, then pharmacologic recommendations. Procedural treatment recommendations are briefly discussed.

NONPHARMACOLOGIC RECOMMENDATIONS
Fitness Plan

Both ACR and AAOS have strong recommendations for some form of fitness. Strong recommendations mean the evidence was high quality for the proposal and that the benefit clearly outweighs the harm.[6,9]

Box 1
Resources for osteoarthritis management

Exercise
  www.YMCA.net
  Fitness Factor www.Fitnessfactor.net
  Core Fitness www.thecore247.com
  Rehab at Work (Physical Therapy) www.rehabatwork.com
  Arthritis Foundation: exercise program, Walk with Ease program, aquatic program www.arthritis.org

Weight control
  Weight Watchers www.weightwatchers.com
  Nutrisystem www.nutrisystem.com

Self-management programs
  Arthritis Foundation www.arthritistoday.org
  CDC arthritis programs www.cdc.gov.arthritis

Tai chi
  Arthritis Foundation www.arthritis.org
  Tai chi videos www.taichiforseniorsvideo.com

Osteoarthritis Management
Core Treatment

Non-pharmacological
Exercise- low-impact aerobic, aquatic, resistance
    Strength training& neuromuscular education
Weight loss (if BMI>25)
Self-management Program(Arthritis Foundation)
Thermal Agents (heat/cold)
Tai Chi

Pharmacological[a]
Oral NSAID +/- PPI
Oral Cox2
Topical capsacin (OTC) or NSAID i.e. Voltaren gel
Acetaminophen (not to exceed 3000mg/day)
Tramadol
Chondrotin Sulfate&/or Glucosamine
    (If no help d/c after 3 mo trial)
CBD oil

LOCATION

Hand
Evaluate ADLs
Instruct in joint protection
Provide assistive devices
Heat modalities
Splint (MCPJ/TMCJ)

Knee

Effusion	No Effusion
Cold therapy	Shoe Insoles[b]
+/- aspiration	Patellar taping[b]
w corticosteroid	

Use mobility aids as needed i.e. cane,
    crutches, or walker
Viscous injection , PRP[c]
    (ref. to orthosurgeon)

Hip
Use mobility aids
    as needed
i.e. cane, crutches,
    or walker

[b]medial wedge shoe insoles for valgus knee OA, subtalar strapped lateral insoles for varus knee, medially directed patellar taping

REFERRAL
Failed conservative treatment with significant functional loss & pain
Refer to Orthopaedic surgeon:
    Send documentation of failed conservative tx modalities
    Anemia work up, Dental evaluation, Sleep apnea study, PT for core strengthening
    Standing AP, Lat & sunrise =knee   AP pelvis & frog leg lateral =Hip

REFUSES REFERRAL OR UNABLE TO BE CLEARED FOR SURGERY
Opioids (Follow American Pain Society/American Academy of Pain Medicine guidelines regarding
    opioid analgesics)
Refer to pain clinic

Fig. 3. Clinical algorithm for nonsurgical management of OA. [a]Comorbid pharmacologic management: NSAIDs use the lowest dose for the shortest duration. Cardiovascular on ASA: acceptable to use most NSAIDs but add proton pump inhibitor (PPI). Do not use ibuprofen (reduces effectiveness of ASA). Do not use cyclooxygenase 2 (Cox-2) inhibitors (celecoxib [Celebrex]). Renal stage IV and V (estimated glomerular filtration rate [eGFR] <30 mL/min) do not use NSAIDs. Evaluate stage III (eGFR 30–59 mL/min) for benefits versus risk. Upper GI bleed within 1 year, use Cox-2 with PPI. History of symptomatic or uncompli-cated ulcer, use NSAID or Cox-2 with PPI. [b]Shoe insoles and patellar taping recommended by ACR guidelines only. [c]Viscous supplementation injections not recommended by AAOS or ACR guidelines. ADL, activities of daily living; AP, anteroposterior; BMI, body mass index; CBD, cannabidiol; OTC, over the counter; MCPJ, metacarpophalangeal joint; PT, physical therapy; TMCJ, trapeziometacarpal joint; tx, treatment. (Copyright © 2020. HealthCom Me-dia. Used with permission. All rights reserved. MyAmericanNurse.com.)

Exercise in the form of low-impact aerobics, aquatic exercise, strength training, and neuromuscular education can be a valuable aid in relieving pain and reducing the impact of progressive disease. Creating a community-based list of local resources for these exercise therapies can be helpful to patients.

Many patients are reluctant to participate in exercise because of pain in a weight-bearing joint.[12,13] Occasionally a physical therapy referral is needed to plot out a plan for an arthritic patient to avoid joint symptoms while strengthening the core. For patients with minimal joint pain and dysfunction, many fitness centers have knowledgeable trainers that can design programs that limit joint irritation and encourage general fitness development. Physical therapy clinics are often associated with or know about local fitness facilities, therefore, when clients are ready, they can be transferred to a fitness facility to continue their core plans, usually for a nominal fee. This system works well and creates continuity of care; it becomes a win-win situation if the patients ever need surgical intervention. They are comfortable with the facility and are usually in better physical shape than if they had not entered into the core fitness plan preoperatively.

An occupational therapy referral may be necessary to address any functional impairments and assist with activities of daily living if indicated. Water aerobics can be encouraged to decrease the pain of weight bearing while increasing muscle strength and fitness. Establishing tone to core muscles, including abdominals, back, and pelvis, is necessary for posture and assists in the stability used in the dynamics of movement. This conditioning can make all the difference in reducing progression of the disease and assist the patient when rehabilitating from surgery, if it becomes indicated.

Weight Loss

Obesity is an issue that affects many people but significantly affects patients with OA as the number 1 preventable risk factor.[4] The general wear and tear of an affected joint is made worse when a patient's body mass index (BMI) exceeds 25. The CDC reports that even a moderate weight loss of 5% can reduce pain and physical disability.[5] Both AAOS and ACR have moderate to strong recommendations for weight loss, especially when combined with exercise.[6,9]

Providers and clinic nurses can encourage patients to maintain a healthy weight. Many caregivers have commented, "Patients know they are overweight so why keep harping on it?"[1] The reason it is mentioned is not to berate the patients but to begin to assist them in making those difficult lifestyle choices that can improve their health and prevent future problems.

Being familiar with the transtheoretical model of change can assist providers to help patients move from one step in the stages of change to another.[14] This process usually takes multiple encounters as the person is helped to focus on the pros of change, becomes informed of the reason for change, and is helped to see how social barriers can be reduced to allow change. Not all patients are ready to make the changes to lose weight initially, but nurses should explore different weight loss options for patients. When combined with exercise, dietary modification can benefit patients with OA significantly.[4,6,13,15]

Some patients have comorbid conditions such as diabetes or hypertension. These conditions warrant specific diet modifications. Therefore, it is important that the nurse be aware of the DASH (Dietary Approaches to Stop Hypertension; https://dashdiet. org/) diet and the American Diabetic Association dietary recommendations (www. diabetes.org).[11] Reviewing healthy diet options, setting goals, and giving written instructions can assist patients who are struggling with their weight. If clinic resources are not sufficient, then knowing the resources in the community is crucial. Dieticians at the local hospital or nursing home may be available for outpatient consultation. Exploring specific programs, such as Weight Watchers (www.weightwatchers.com) or dietary sites available online can help give patients hope. It is important to help patients set achievable goals with the long-term aim of reducing pain and increasing function. Most patients respond to nurses who develop a relationship and care enough to help with dietary recommendations.

Self-Management

Self-management is an area that is strongly recommended by both the ACR and AAOS guidelines.[6,9] Studies have shown that persons who are active in their own care reach goals and are able to sustain behavioral changes that improve quality of life.[15]

The Arthritis Foundation and the CDC have multiple self-management programs available for patients with OA.[4,5] Nurses can easily locate the site and assist patients in accessing this information. The self-management programs vary from 6-week courses to phone follow-up and workshops through the Arthritis Foundation.[4] Several studies showed statistically significant differences in pain, stiffness, and mobility when patients engaged in these programs. These programs are led by nurses, physical therapists, occupational therapist, health coaches, and educators.[4,5]

Many patients participate in online programs (see **Box 1**). One in 4 Americans has an impairment that affects their ability to move. A helpful AAOS Web site is www.anationinmotion.org. This site has patient success stories, a motivational game called I Can, and a place for people to upload their own stories. It is very encouraging and helps people relate to one another, especially with mobility issues. The National Council on Aging (www.ncoa.org/) has multiple helpful guides for patients on how to manage chronic illness, exercise, and even weight management, and it also has online courses in self-management. The CDC (www.cdc.org) Web site has several recommendations for physical activity and self-management education programs, with several more in development. Do not "reinvent the wheel," but encourage clinic nurses to break out and be assertive in their care; they might even start a patient class to assist with self-management.

Mobility Aids, Bracing/Taping, and Insoles

The use of mobility aids when needed is recommended by both AAOS and ACR. There was not enough evidence for the use of knee braces from AAOS, which made their recommendation inconclusive. The only recommendations for bracing by the ACR were for hand OA. Only the ACR conditionally recommends patellar taping and wedged shoe insoles. Insoles may be indicated for patients with medial compartment OA, and laterally wedged insoles with a subtalar strap are recommended for lateral compartment OA.[6,9]

Thermal Agents

AAOS did not address the use of thermal agents in their guidelines, but the ACR had conditional recommendations for the use of these agents.[6,9] The recommendation to use ice is based on the antiinflammatory effect. If the joint is inflamed, then encourage the use of ice. In contrast, heat helps with stiffness but should be avoided if a synovial reaction is occurring. Heat is primarily used for pain relief in the form of paraffin wax baths for patients with severe OA of the hands. Instruct patients to avoid lying on a heating pad, and to watch for burns.

Practical ideas for ice application:

1. Use a bag of peas from the freezer for better compliance. This method is easier and less expensive than some alternatives. Inform the patients to use the iced peas for only 15 to 20 minutes at a time and not directly on skin, and do not eat the peas.

2. Homemade ice packs can be made using three-quarters of a cup of alcohol with 3.5 cups of water and a few drops of food coloring, if desired. Place the liquid in a ziplock bag, tape well, and freeze.

Tai Chi

Tai chi is a graceful form of exercise, sometimes described as meditation in motion.[4] It is a low-impact physical exercise that most patients tolerate and enjoy. It provides constant motion while assisting with strength and balance. It is generally safe for anyone, especially for those with a chronic illness. The AAOS had no discussion of tai chi in their recommendations but the ACR touted the benefits for knee OA, although not enough evidence was available to make a recommendation for hip OA.[6,9]

The Arthritis Foundation and Mayo Clinic are strong supporters of tai chi as a means to assist patients in developing core body strength, improving movement, and reducing pain.[4,16] A study in Boston, Massachusetts, showed significant benefits for people with all types of arthritis. Those who participated in a tai chi program had significant pain relief, less stiffness, and better ability to manage daily living. The participants felt better about their overall wellness, and had improved balance.[4] Several resources are available for tai chi. The Arthritis Foundation has a tai chi program as well as videos to buy for home use.[4] Some local yoga studios, spas, and even the YMCA have classes. Tai chi videos can also be found on the Internet for free (YouTube).

PHARMACOLOGIC RECOMMENDATIONS

AAOS had strong recommendations and the ACR had conditional recommendations for the use of NSAIDs, oral or topical, or tramadol (Ultram) for symptomatic patients.[6,9]

Health care providers used NSAIDs in large doses for many years, then they changed to avoiding NSAIDs because of concern for cardiovascular and gastrointestinal (GI) side effects. Research now shows that NSAIDs are safe when used in the appropriate patients, for the shortest amount of time, and at the lowest effective dose. CDC reported NSAID-related GI bleeding as the 14th leading cause of death in the United States in 2011.[5] Using naproxen sodium or ibuprofen over the counter (OTC)can provide effective relief for many patients while reducing the threat of side effects. If a patient is on low-dose acetylsalicylic acid (ASA) for cardioprotection, then concomitant use of ibuprofen should be avoided because it may render the ASA ineffective.[9,17] Occasionally some patients want a prescription for these medications because they may be cheaper with insurance coverage.

NSAID use with a proton pump inhibitor (PPI) such as omeprazole (Prilosec) OTC can help to reduce GI toxicity. H_2 receptor blockers are not as effective because they do not give significant relief of gastric ulcers, only duodenal ulcers. The exception is a double dose of famotidine (Pepcid) twice a day, which has been shown to reduce duodenal and gastric ulcers with long-term NSAID use.[18]

The oral cyclooxygenase 2 (Cox-2) inhibitor, celecoxib (Celebrex) is the only one currently available, but may be expensive. This drug is a good option in combination with a PPI if a patient has had an upper GI bleed within a year.[9] With any history of a GI bleed, celecoxib (Celebrex) alone may be adequate.[9]

Remember to adequately evaluate the patient's renal function before starting an NSAID. If renal disease is stage 3, glomerular filtration rate (GFR) 30 to 59 mL/min, then use with caution. If the renal disease is stage 4 to 5, GFR less than 30 mL/min, then do not use NSAIDs.[9]

Topical NSAIDs are available; the most accessible is topical capsaicin and its use is supported by both the AAOS and ACR.[6,9] Topical diclofenac gel (Voltaren) is successful in many patients and can be used up to 4 times a day on sore, painful joints with minimal side effects. It is inexpensive at around $45 for a 1-g tube but requires a prescription.

Acetaminophen (Tylenol) was used first line for a few years following the increase in GI side effects of NSAIDs. Now the AAOS categorizes it as having inconclusive evidence as to the benefit.[6] They found that the use of acetaminophen (Tylenol) had no benefit compared with a placebo. The ACR only conditionally recommends its use.[9] Patient preference should have a substantial influencing role. New pharmaceutical recommendations establish a maximum dose of 3000 mg/d.[6]

Inconclusive evidence was found for opioid and pain patch use by both groups.[6,9] They both recommended opioid use only for those symptomatic patients who have failed conservative treatment modalities and are either not able or unwilling candidates for total joint arthroplasty. Then the provider should follow the American Pain Society guidelines and refer the patient to a pain clinic.

AAOS and ACR cannot recommend chondroitin sulfate and/or glucosamine, because there is strong evidence that there are no clinically significant benefits compared with placebo.[6,9] Some patients like it and find it effective. If a patient expresses an interest in trying these supplements, then suggest a 3-month trial. If the trial is not effective, then stop taking it.

A new OTC medication that is gaining acceptance is cannabidiol (CBD) oil. Neither AAOS nor ACR spoke to this new trend.[6,9] It is hoped that this may be discussed in upcoming guidelines. Many patients are stating that they find good relief for arthritic pain while using oral or topical CBD oil. Patients should be aware that the US Food and Drug Administration (FDA) does not regulate CBD oil so the guarantee of consistent potency and purity in the capsules is variable. If patients want to try it, they need to be educated. The oil comes from hemp, which is the *Cannabis sativa* plant. This form does not have the tetrahydrocannabinol component, which, in marijuana, can get people "high." If patients want to try CBD oil, then recommend they purchase it from a reputable pharmacist who is familiar with different brands and potency. Always use the lowest dose possible. If it is not effective, stop using it.[19]

PROCEDURAL TREATMENTS

Corticosteroids, viscous supplementation, stem cells, and platelet-rich plasma intra-articular injections are discussed in the guidelines. Prolotherapy, defined later in this article, was not covered. Many of these intra-articular treatments have come into more prevalent use since the guidelines were introduced. It is hoped that these treatments will be addressed in the new guidelines.

Corticosteroids

The oldest and most common intra-articular treatment is cortisone injections. Many patients begin serial injections 3 to 4 times a year to obtain relief from OA joint pain. If the patient has an effusion, some providers aspirate the fluid then instill cortisone into the joint for relief. AAOS and ACR both found inconclusive evidence that cortisone injections help.[6,9] The problem is that there were not enough studies in 2012 and 2013 to support a strong recommendation for use. In the 2017 *AAOS Surgical Guidelines for the Hip*, recommendations supported intra-articular corticosteroids to improve function and reduce pain in hip OA.

Viscous Supplementation

Viscous supplementation injections (hyaluronic acid) are promoted to maintain synovial fluid viscosity and support articular cartilage shock absorption. AAOS and ACR cannot recommend their use.[6,9] There is strong evidence that there are no clinically significant benefits compared with placebo. This recommendation was based on lack of efficacy and not on potential harm. AAOS recommendations in 2017 for the hip continued to show that there was no significant improvement compared with a placebo in using viscous supplementation injections.[8]

More studies will be done to ascertain whether the financial cost with minimal improvement justifies its use. Some patients like it and find it effective.

Prolotherapy

"Prolotherapy is an injection that contains a potential irritant, such as a dextrose solution. The irritant is thought to trigger the body's healing response."[20] This procedure has gained momentum in the current climate but there are not enough studies to support positive outcomes from the procedure.[4] It is not covered by insurance or Medicare.

Stem Cells

The goal of injecting stem cells into arthritic joints is to regrow cartilage. A comprehensive review by Zhao and colleagues[23] in 2018 revealed that regenerative medicine technologies such as the use of stem cells are promising in the treatment of OA of the knee. However, the main concern is about the lack of standardization of the available stem cells.[21] Unless there is participation in a clinical research study, pure stem cells are not available in the United States. The only other source of cells is a mix of a variety of cells. Without pure cells, it is difficult to determine whether treatments contain enough stem cells for consistent results. AAOS guidelines were unable to recommend for or against their use in OA.[6]

Platelet-Rich Plasma

The aim of platelet-rich plasma (PRP) intra-articular injection is to produce a cartilage matrix while also decreasing the inflammatory response. The procedure includes drawing the patient's blood, centrifuging it to remove red blood cells, then administering the platelets into the joint. The platelets are usually activated in a variety of methods. AAOS guidelines were unable to recommend for or against its use in OA.[6] Once again, there were not enough quality studies available. However, several systematic reviews and meta-analyses have been reported since the guidelines were published. In 2019, a review of current evidence for PRP in OA by Gato-Calvo and colleagues[24] stated that the randomized controlled trials reviewed seem to be favorable for the use of PRP. These injections seem to improve pain scores more than other intra-articular injections. The results were more favorable in patients in early stages of OA, but the overall evidence is low. Therefore, the treatment is still under debate.[22]

REFERRAL CRITERIA

So when should you refer a patient? Is this all that needs to be done? Refer the patient and then primary care is finished? No. This is the time to turn up the heat! A referral is made when the patient is not quite ready for a total joint arthroplasty, although it may be inevitable. This referral should be a trigger to take stock in the patient's general health and begin an intentional plan of preparation. Work with orthopedics to get patients in shape while waiting for surgery, especially when cortisone or viscous supplementation injections give pain relief. This time is the perfect opportunity to make a difference in the patient's treatment plan and outcomes.

If the referral includes obtaining radiographs, always get standing anteroposterior (AP), lateral, and sunrise views to thoroughly evaluate the knee. This evaluation saves the patient money and radiation. If it is a hip, get AP pelvis and frog-leg lateral views of the hip for the best evaluation of OA in the joint.

Once OA has progressed to the point where surgery is inevitable, the nurse can help prepare the patient. There are no direct guidelines from AAOS or ACR as to what preoperative evaluations should be performed. However, the following suggestions are based on the frequency of postoperative complications and evaluations. Ways to help avoid these issues include creating the best possible health, including weight, attitude, and positive general health markers such as adequate hematocrit (Hct) and hemoglobin (Hgb), normalized blood glucose, albumin, vitamin D, and renal function levels. All of these can help ensure that the patient is in the best possible condition before surgery. When obstructive sleep apnea (OSA), dental conditions, and anemia are evaluated before surgery, postoperative complications can be minimized.

Anemia is a complicating factor postoperatively because of surgical blood loss. Assessment of Hct and Hgb is a good way to begin evaluation of potential surgical patients. If the Hct and Hgb levels are low, then further evaluation is necessary to determine whether the patient has iron deficiency and can be treated with iron. If the Hct and Hgb levels are too low, then referral to a hematologist may be necessary. If these preoperative evaluations are not done until scheduling of the surgery, then the procedure may have to be postponed in order to get the patient in optimal shape for the elective procedure. There is no need to wait until an arthroplasty is scheduled to make these evaluations. Primary care nurses can be proactive and assist patients with evaluation of these conditions under the direction of the primary health care provider.

Primary care nurses can educate patients with OA on the need for regular dental care. In the past, prophylactic antibiotics were prescribed for patients who had undergone prosthetic joint replacement surgeries. In January 2015, the American Dental Association released clinical practice guidelines based on a systematic review from 2014. The review states, "In general, for patients with prosthetic joint implants, prophylactic antibiotics are not recommended prior to dental procedures to prevent prosthetic joint infection."[23] Although postoperative care has changed, preoperative considerations to make sure a patient has no potential for infection caused by poor dentition is still appropriate.

Another high-risk comorbidity is OSA; postoperative atelectasis is higher in persons with OSA. "Ideally, identification of patients with OSA, whether adherent or nonadherent to therapy, and those with suspected OSA should take place well in advance of elective surgery to allow time for potential evaluation and management of OSA preoperatively."[24] Therefore preoperative evaluations are indicated if the patient is obese; snores; and has excessive daytime sleepiness, morning headaches, and periods of breathing cessation. If a patient requires a continuous positive airway pressure machine, then the patient should be asked to bring it to the hospital for postoperative recovery.

A current trend in OA evaluation recommendations is to evaluate patients for osteoporosis. Long-term complications, from lack of bone density around the tip of the prosthesis once the arthroplasty is performed, contribute to pain and loosening of the prosthesis. Therefore, it is suggested, at a minimum, to evaluate these patients using the Fracture Risk Assessment Tool (FRAX) (www.sheffield.ac.uk/FRAX/tool.aspx).[25] Vitamin D levels can be checked and evaluated.[25] If the level is low, proceed to a DEXA (dual-energy x-ray absorptiometry) scan.[26] Based on the results, a patient may benefit from anabolic medications to rebuild new bone. These medications can be used for 2 to 24 months before surgery and followed up with bisphosphonates as indicated.

TEAMWORK

A large percentage of patients come to office visits with 3 or more complaints. The visit time is not getting any longer, but more listening, especially at the beginning of the visit, can help narrow down the plan and ensure the patient feels heard. This approach also eliminates the "Oh, I had one more question" when the provider is leaving the room. Use the clinic team; encourage nurses or medical assistants to use their ability to assist with the objective. The provider should share with the team what is important. Most nurses ask the history of present illness and document this in the computer, so make sure lifestyle areas are discussed and documented. Most of these patients are there to be seen for other chronic illnesses. While treating diabetes mellitus with diet and exercise, a simple discussion of how that will affect their OA can be added. Core strengthening, weight loss, and self-management protocols could be initiated by clinic personnel if they are educated and encouraged to do so. Always address weight control and physical activity.

There is no need to stop care for OA just because the patient is referred to a specialist. patients still need weight loss, core strengthening, and preoperative proactive care. Long term, explore the use of self-management programs for the average patients with OA. Continue to look at local referral sources, always thinking of financial limitations. Teach nurses to be proactive within their scope of practice, such as weight loss, exercise options, and self-help management programs.

SUMMARY

My friend, after having her total joint, joined a local gym, is trying to lose weight, and is working on her general fitness level. She is a retired nurse and has plans. If only someone had taken the time to encourage her to take care of herself earlier, retirement may be just a little more enjoyable.

This is too big a problem for an already busy practitioner to tackle alone. The care of OA takes a systems approach. NPs who want to provide increased support of their patients' self-management are advised to address 3 areas: structure their patient-provider interactions to include goal-setting and problem-solving strategies, make office system changes, and provide self-management education by linking patients to community or online programs.

Have a vision and make it your mission to treat chronic illnesses in an intentional way. The patients will appreciate the comprehensive, intentional care given to make their lives easier and more productive. Do not let your patients be the ones who say, "If only someone had told me."

ACKNOWLEDGMENTS

I would like to acknowledge the assistance of Alena Lester, DNP, APRN, FNP-C, ONP-C expert and content reviewer.

DISCLOSURE

The author has nothing to disclose.

REFERENCES

1. Pearson S. Implementing evidenced-based practice guidelines for the management of osteoarthritis: an assessment in primary care. [thesis]. Columbus,(MS): Mississippi University for Women; 2013.
2. Barbour KE, Helmick CG, Boring M, et al. Vital signs: prevalence of doctor-diagnosed arthritis and arthritis-attributable activity limitation—United States, 2013–2015. MMWR Morb Mortal Wkly Rep 2017;66:246–53.
3. United States Census Bureau. Quick Facts 2018. Available at: https://www.census.gov/quickfacts/fact/table/ca,ms/PST045218. Accessed January 20, 2019.
4. Arthritis Foundation. About Arthritis. Available at: https://www.arthritis.org/about-arthritis/understanding-arthritis/what-is-arthritis.php https://www.arthritis.org/living-with-arthritis/exercise/workouts/other-activities/tai-chi-arthritis.php https://www.arthritis.org/living-with-arthritis/treatments/medication/drug-types/other/prolotherapy-knee-oa.php. Accessed December 17, 2018.
5. **CDC. Available at: https://www.cdc.gov/arthritis/data_statistics/national-statistics.html https://www.cdc.gov/healthyweight/losing_weight/index.html https://www.cdc.gov/learnmorefeelbetter/programs/arthritis.htm.
6. American Academy of Orthopaedic Surgeons. Treatment of osteoarthritis of the knee evidence-based guideline. 2nd edition. Rosemont (IL): American Academy of Orthopaedic Surgeons; 2013.
7. American Academy of Orthopaedic Surgeons. Surgical management of osteoarthritis of the knee: evidence-based clinical practice guidelines. Rosemont (IL): American Academy of Orthopaedic Surgeons; 2015.
8. American Academy of Orthopaedic Surgeons. Management of osteoarthritis of the hip. Rosemont (IL): American Academy of Orthopaedic Surgeons; 2017. Available at: https://www.aaos.org/uploadedFiles/PreProduction/Quality/Guidelines_and_Reviews/OA Hip CPG_1.5.18.pdf. Accessed February 12, 2019.
9. Hochberg M, Altman R, April K, et al. American College of Rheumatology 2012 recommendations for the use of nonpharmacologic and pharmacologic therapies in osteoarthritis of the hand, hip, and knee. Arthritis Care Res 2012;64(4):465–74.
10. Beckman HB, Frankel RM. The effect of physician behavior on the collection of data. Ann Intern Med 1984;101:692–6.
11. Hurley M. Self-management for osteoarthritis: where have we escaped to? Rheumatology 2018;57(3). https://doi.org/10.1093/rheumatology/key075.077.
12. A randomized, controlled trial of total knee replacement. NEJM. (n.d.). Available at: https://www.nejm.org/doi/10.1056/NEJMoa1505467?url_ver=Z39.88-2003&rfr_id=ori%3Arid%3Acrossref.org&rfr_dat=cr_pub%3Dwww.ncbi.nlm.nih.gov. Accessed October 9, 2018.
13. Messier SP, Mihalko SL, Legault C, et al. Effects of intensive diet and exercise on knee joint loads, inflammation, and clinical outcomes among overweight and obese adults with knee osteoarthritis: the IDEA randomized clinical trial. JAMA 2013;310(12):1263–73.
14. Prochaska J, Redding A, Evers K. The transtheoretical model and stages of change. In: Glanz K, Rimer B, Viswanath K, editors. Health behavior theory, research, and practice. 5th edition. San Francisco (CA): Jossey-Bass; 2015. p. 125–48 [Chapter: 7].
15. Available at: https://www.mayoclinic.org/healthy-lifestyle/stress-management/indepth/tai-chi/art-20045184. Accessed June 25, 2019.
16. Fletcher J. What is prolotherapy and what is it used to treat? Medical News Today 2017. Available at: https://www.medicalnewstoday.com/articles/320330.php.

17. Sollecito TP, Abt E, Lockhart PB, et al. The use of prophylactic antibiotics prior to dental procedures in patients with prosthetic joints: evidence-based clinical practice guideline for dental practitioners–a report of the American Dental Association Council on Scientific Affairs. J Am Dent Assoc 2015;146(1):11–6.e8.
18. Tuskey A, Peura D. The use of H2 antagonists in treating and preventing NSAID-induced mucosal damage. Arthritis Res Ther 2013;15(Suppl 3):S6.
19. Chung F. Society of Anesthesia and Sleep Medicine Guidelines on preoperative screening and assessment of adult patients with obstructive sleep apnea. Anesth Analg 2016;123(2):452–73.
20. Pearson S. Proactive intervention for osteoarthritis. Am Nurse Today 2015;10(8): 2162–8629.
21. Hohlfeld T, Saxena A, Schrör K, et al. High on treatment platelet reactivity against aspirin by non-steroidal anti-inflammatory drugs—pharmacological mechanisms and clinical relevance. Thromb Haemost 2013;109. https://doi.org/10.1160/TH12-07-532.
22. Rath L. CBD oil: should you try it for arthritis symptoms? Arthritis Foundation. Available at: https://www.arthritis.org/living-with-arthritis/treatments/natural/supplements-herbs/cannabidiol-oil.php. Accessed May 17, 2019.
23. Zhao L, Kaye AD, Abd-Elsayed A. Stem cells for the treatment of knee osteoarthritis: a comprehensive review. Pain Physician 2018;21(3):229–42.
24. Gato-Calvo L, Magalhaes J, Ruiz-Romero C, et al. Platelet-rich plasma in osteoarthritis treatment: review of current evidence. Ther Adv Chronic Dis 2019. https://doi.org/10.1177/2040622319825567.
25. Pfotenhauer KM, Shubrook JH. Vitamin D deficiency, its role in health and disease, and current supplementation recommendations. J Am Osteopath Assoc 2017;117(5):301.
26. Papaioannou A, Morin S, Cheung AM, et al, for the Scientific Advisory Council of Osteoporosis Canada. 2010 clinical practice guidelines for the diagnosis and management of osteoporosis in Canada: summary. CMAJ 2010;182(17): 1864–73.

Innovations in Care of the Elderly Hip Fracture Patient; a Nightmare No More

Kari L. Baerwald Erickson, BAN, RN, ONC

KEYWORDS

- Hip fracture • Fragility fracture • Clinical pathway • Multidisciplinary • Osteoporosis

KEY POINTS

- Hip fracture in the elderly is a problem occurring in communities.
- The most common type of hip fracture in the elderly is a low-trauma fracture, often called a fragility fracture.
- Fragility fractures are caused by osteoporosis.
- Comorbidities contribute to complications and increased length of stay for elderly hip fracture patients.
- Comprehensive hip fracture programs lead to best outcomes after surgery.

INTRODUCTION

Hip fractures that occur in the elderly population continue to be a growing problem in communities. In this article, the elderly are defined as patients who are 65 years and older. In this particular population, patients often have multiple comorbidities. These comorbidities cause challenges for a patient's optimization preoperatively and throughout the continuum of care. Mortality rates among this population are 30% higher within the first year after fracture. Many more experience major loss of function and mobility. Hip fracture incidence is likely to increase as the population ages and lives longer. Medical facilities are under pressure to reduce costs and improve outcomes.[1]

This article focuses on the epidemiology, prevalence, and trends of hip fractures in the elderly worldwide. In addition, a typical care pathway, sharing best practices and innovative nursing care strategies with anticipated outcomes, is discussed.

EPIDEMIOLOGY

Epidemiologic data vary between countries, but it is globally estimated that hip fractures affect approximately 18% of women and 6% of men. Thus, the global number of

Orthopedics, Sanford Medical Center Fargo, 1720 University Drive South, Fargo, ND 58122, USA
E-mail address: kari.erickson@sanfordhealth.org

Nurs Clin N Am 55 (2020) 149–161
https://doi.org/10.1016/j.cnur.2020.02.010
0029-6465/20/© 2020 Elsevier Inc. All rights reserved.

hip fractures is expected to increase from 1.26 million in 1990 to 4.5 million by the year 2050.[2,3] **Fig. 1** visually displays the projected number of osteoporotic hip fractures, according to the National Osteoporosis Foundation. Osteoporotic hip fractures often cause the low-trauma, fragility fracture. Rapid rise of the osteoporotic hip fracture population may be compromised by focusing on prevention. Prevention is made possible by the treatment of osteoporosis and fall risk. Nonmodifiable factors (such as age, race, and sex), however, also affect hip fracture incidence.[2]

OSTEOPOROSIS

Bone is living and growing tissue essential to protect and support the body. Bones constantly and continually remodel and renew to fit the body's needs. Bone cells, known as osteoblasts, build bone, whereas osteoclasts dissolve bone. The equilibrium between the 2 processes, bone building and bone dissolving, is affected negatively with age. Through the aging process, the rate of building new bone slows down, causing bone loss to occur more quickly than bone building. Certain diseases, medical procedures, and even certain medications can cause bone loss as well. Osteoporosis means "porous bone." Osteoporosis often is called a silent disease because patients cannot feel bones weakening. Breaking a bone often is the first sign of osteoporosis[4] (**Table 1**).

HIP FRACTURE TYPES

Fig. 2 displays the normal anatomy of the hip. The most common hip fracture types are femoral neck fracture (**Fig. 3**) and intertrochanteric hip fracture (**Fig. 4**).

Femoral neck fracture (see **Fig. 3**) has been known to cause the most risk for complications preoperatively, because it occurs closer to the hip joint. By being

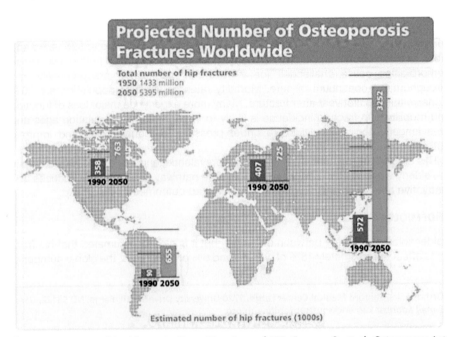

Fig. 1. Fracture world-wide projection. (*Courtesy of* IOF. Cooper C, et al. Osteoporos Int. 1992;2(6):285-9. Hip fractures in the elderly: a world-wide projection; with permission.)

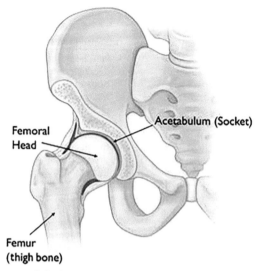

Femoral Head

Acetabulum (Socket)

Femur (thigh bone)

Fig. 2. Normal anatomy of the hip.

closer to the hip joint, this type of fracture poses risk for cutting off blood supply to the femur. Intertrochanteric hip fracture (see **Fig. 4**) happens further away from the hip joint, causing less risk of interrupting the blood supply.

With either fracture, repair is most often necessary to establish stabilization of the hip. By stabilizing the hip joint, through surgical intervention, patients have a greater chance to return to their preoperative functional state.

CAUSES OF HIP FRACTURE

In relation to osteoporosis and the 2 most common types of hip fractures, a fall is the most common reason for a hip fracture among the elderly.[5] It is known that osteoporosis causes weak and thinned bones. Something as basic as a fall from standing height would cause a break to an already weakened, soft, thin bone.

Upon epidemiologic data review, prevalence of hip fractures occurs primarily among women. As women age, hormones fluctuate, causing less estrogen to be produced by their bodies. Estrogen helps maintain the strength and density, or thickness, of bones. Women who have estrogen deficiency can develop osteoporosis of their bones.

RISKS FOR HIP FRACTURE

A person with osteoporosis is at risk for a hip fracture. Other conditions that may increase the risk even more include

- Excessive alcohol consumption
- Lack of physical activity
- Low body weight
- Poor nutrition, including a diet low on calcium and vitamin D
- Gender
- Tall stature
- Vision problems
- Thinking problems, such as dementia

Table 1
Hip fracture programs

Conventional Hip Fracture Program	Optimized Hip Fracture Program
1. The primary choice of pain treatment was subcutaneous injections or tablets of morphine, 2.5–5 mg as needed. After surgery, tablets of sustained-release morphine, 10–20 mg, twice a day, were used. Supplementary pain treatment: acetaminophen tablets, 1 g, 4 times a day, and ibuprofen, 400 mg, 3 times a day.	1. Pain treatment consisted of a femoral nerve catheter block. Bolus injection of bupivacaine, 20 mL (5 mg/mL). Maintenance dose bupivacaine, 20 mL (2.5 mg/mL), 4 times a day. If adverse events occurred, the dose was reduced to 10 mL, 4 times a day. Supplementary pain treatment: tablet acetaminophen, 1 g, 4 times a day, and eventually tablet ibuprofen, 400 mg, 3 times a day.
2. Assessment by an anesthesiologist, planning of fluid therapy, preoperative blood samples in the admission ward after the medical record had been obtained	2. Assessment by anesthesiologist, planning of fluid therapy, preoperative blood samples in the ED
3. The ED physician evaluated radiographs after the patient had returned to the ED from the department of radiology.	3. The radiographer evaluated the radiographs. A positive radiograph for hip fracture led to direct transfer to the specialized hip fracture ward unit.
4. Before surgery, the patient entered an admission ward unit and after surgery was transferred to 1 of 5 possible ward units.	4. Before and after surgery, the patient stayed on a specialized hip fracture ward unit.
5 Nutrition therapy for selected patients only. No food and drinks allowed within 6 h before surgery.	5. Water, lemonade, and carbohydrate-enriched drinks were allowed until 2 h before surgery. Normal diet was allowed until 6 h before surgery.
6. Assessment of nutritional status if the patient recently had lost weight or had a low body mass index (<23 kg/m^2) at admission	6 All patients had an assessment of nutritional status at the admission, and ,if necessary, nutrition therapy was started. All patients were offered high-protein or 12.5% carbohydrate-rich drinks.
7. Oxygen therapy only to patients with pneumonia or acute respiratory failure	7. Oxygen therapy, 2 L/min, through a nasal catheter when resting and during the first 4 nights
8. Suspicion of urinary retention resulted in single catheterizations and, if it continued, a catheter for a few days.	8. If urinary retention was suspected, an ultrasonic bladder scan was performed. The first urinary retention resulted in a single catheterization and the second in continuous catheterization for 1–2 d.

From Robertson, B D and Robertson, T J. Postoperative Delirium After Hip Fracture. Journal of Bone and Joint Surgery. 2016 Sep; 88(9): 2060-2068. Accessed March 30, 2019. https://doi.org/10.2106/JBJS.F.00049

- Physical problems
- Medicines that cause bone loss
- Cigarette smoking
- Living in an assisted-care facility
- Increased risk for falls, related to conditions, such as weakness, disability, or unsteady gait[5]

PREVENTING A HIP FRACTURE

Reversing any of the modifiable risk factors is key in helping to decrease the risk of hip fracture. Trends of hip fractures worldwide will continue to increase, as projected in

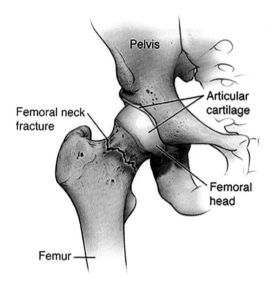

Fig. 3. Femoral neck fracture.

Fig. 1, if steps to prevent their occurrence do not happen. Nurses have the opportunity to educate those who have had a hip fracture, and those at risk, to make modifiable lifestyle changes. Some examples to help educate patients and their families are as follows.

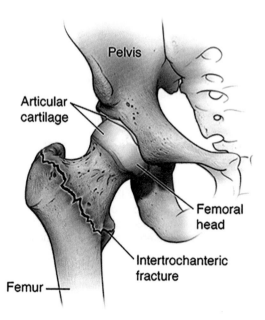

Fig. 4. Intertrochanteric hip fracture.

- Limiting alcohol consumption
- Increasing physical activity as able
  - Walking if able, making sure to walk on a flat open surface with good walking shoes
- Maintaining healthy body weight
  - Seeking help from a provider for weight gain or weight loss concerns
- Increasing calcium and vitamin D into diet
  - Dairy products and leafy green vegetables are good examples
  - Taking calcium and vitamin D supplements, if recommended by a provider
- Quitting smoking
  - Asking for help; using online sources or referrals from a provider
- Limiting risk for falls
  - Using an assistive device, such as a walker, if needed
  - Clearing clutter in living spaces
  - Picking up scatter rugs to avoid tripping
  - Having well-lit rooms and hallways
  - Keeping pets away from pathways
  - Using handrails when climbing stairs
- Talking to a provider about ways to enhance bone health

HIP FRACTURE PROGRAMS

A comprehensive hip fracture program, fast-track hip fracture program, and geriatric hip fracture program all are ways of naming the coordination of care for this patient population. This coordination of care, under any of these programs, can be defined through a multidisciplinary clinical care pathway.

The goal of the clinical care pathway is to optimize the patient throughout the continuum of care by expediting an emergency department (ED) to operating room (OR) process, reducing hospital postoperative complications, and enhancing coordination of care. A clinical pathway is a sequential plan of care that involves a structured multidisciplinary approach to address a specific health care problem, according to evidence-based guidelines.[6] In cases of elderly hip fracture patients, this standardized program is initiated most often in an ED, as the patient's primary point of entry.

Developing programs are adding a prehospital phase in this plan of care. Reaching out to involve emergency medical services (EMS) personnel can be beneficial to patients and their outcomes.

HIP FRACTURE CARE PATHWAY AND NURSING CARE STRATEGIES
Emergency Medical Services

An official diagnosis of hip fracture does not occur until a radiograph is viewed by a provider. If a hip fracture is suspected in the field, however, EMS personnel may initiate an approved protocol. This protocol most often includes stabilization for transfer and initial treatment of pain. The EMS staff are essential in gathering information from the patient, family, and even the environment of the incident.

Emergency Department

Unless a patient is a direct admission to an inpatient nursing unit, the ED is the main entry of the hip fracture patient to the hospital. Following the transition of care from EMS, a standard guideline or order set for the patient on arrival is essential. Points of care:

Assessment of cognition

With advanced age, hip fracture patients need baseline assessment of cognition. Dementia is a common concern with this population. Whether arriving from a skilled facility with a specific diagnosis, or assessing a patient and speaking with family members to document current baseline characteristics are important. The importance of the current level of cognition comes into play when looking for signs of delirium, specifically in the postoperative phase.

The most frequent complication associated with hip fracture in elderly patients is postoperative delirium. Delirium consists of a "disturbance of consciousness...with reduced ability to focus, sustain, or shift attention."[7] The diagnostic criteria for delirium have been established by the American Psychiatric Association and are listed in **Box 1**. It is important to be aware of, and to use, these criteria because many of the signs and symptoms of delirium also are associated with conditions, such as dementia, depression, and psychosis.[7]

Pain

Presenting by crying out in pain, or even denying pain, the elderly hip fracture patient can be challenging to assess. This devastating condition of hip fracture leads to pain and immobilization, which must be treated during the preoperative phase.

Careful attention is given to the pain that a patient is experiencing because inappropriate pain control favors delirium, and those with delirium may receive inadequate analgesia.[8]

Optimized programs today initiate pain relief via nerve blocks. This block, administered in the ED, provides overall pain relief when combined with scheduled intravenous or oral analgesia. If needed, this block also can be left in postoperatively several days and is managed by anesthesia.

Nutrition

At the time of hospital admission, a geriatric patient with hip fracture may be clinically malnourished and dehydrated. Recent studies have shown that patients with hip fracture have a higher incidence of protein-energy malnutrition than age-matched controls, which can contribute to the development of postoperative wound complications, infection, and mortality.[9,10] **Table 1** gives reference to offering carbohydrate-enriched drinks up to 2 hours before surgery.

Enhanced recovery after surgery (ERAS) is the buzzwords in elective surgery cases but also can be used in populations, such as hip fracture. The ED can initiate nutrition by giving a preoperative drink loaded with carbohydrates. Often, clear liquids are allowed until

---

Box 1
Diagnostic criteria for delirium

Disturbance in consciousness (impaired ability to focus, sustain, or shift attention).

Change in cognition (memory impairment, disorientation, or language disturbance) or perceptual disturbance (misinterpretations, illusions, or hallucinations).

The disturbance develops over a short period of time and fluctuates during the course of the day.

There is laboratory or clinical evidence that the delirium state is caused by the direct physiologic consequences of a general medical condition.

Adapted from Lawlor PG, Bush SH. Delirium diagnosis, screening and management. Curr Opin Support Palliat Care 2014;8(3):286–95. doi: 10.1097/SPC.0000000000000062.

2 hours before surgery. Depending on medical optimization and timing, ERAS is something that could be initiated in the ED along with assessment of nutritional status.

Skin integrity

A head-to-toe skin assessment is performed on admission. Special care should be given to the pressure points, in particular the coccyx and heels. Skin protection to these areas during time of immobility is important to prevent shearing and damage to skin integrity. Application of skin protection to these areas along with frequent turning of patients preoperatively is an example of best nursing care practice.

Additional points of care

- Laboratory work
- Radiographs
- Electrocardiogram (EKG)
- Urinary assessment and catheter placement
- Monitoring of intake and output
- Other points of care related to a patient's individual history

Case management has an opportunity to establish rapport and initiate conversations with patients and their families. Part of this visit is to start the discussion for care beyond the hospital. Emphasis can be placed on the fact that the hospital is really the first step in the recovery. Further rehabilitation often is needed after the immediate postoperative recovery time, requiring a transition to another facility. A detailed assessment and profile to transitional facilities may be started at this time.

Table 1 outlines the conventional hip fracture program, compared with the optimized hip fracture programs seen today.[7] This table provides a visual summary of the initial discussion thus far in the article for optimized hip fracture programs.

INDICATIONS FOR SURGERY

Surgery is indicated for most patients with hip fracture. Surgical repair often provides better and more rapid pain control and improved mobility. A decision to pursue operative management needs to be considered carefully in the context of benefits and risks of orthopedic surgery, symptom management, and a patient's life expectancy. In patients with life-limiting diseases, such as advanced dementia, patient-centered comprehensive interdisciplinary palliative and hospice care without concurrent operative management may be a more suitable model of care.[11]

TIMING OF SURGERY

The timing of surgery in patients with hip fracture, although ultimately set by the surgeon, often is dictated by the preoperative medical evaluation.[11] Evidence shows the following as guidelines to help the goal of returning patients to their prefunctional status:

- Perform early surgery (within 24 hours) in patients who are medically stable and do not have significant comorbid illness.
- Early surgery may reduce pain and decrease length of stay.
- Whenever possible, surgery should not be delayed beyond 72 hours.

OPERATING ROOM

Patients enter the OR suite when surgically optimized. When possible, the use of spinal anesthesia works well with the elderly population by limiting postoperative complications. General anesthesia in the elderly has been known to cause an increase in postoperative delirium, pneumonia, risk for pulmonary embolism, and deep vein thrombosis.[12]

Research shows that having a dedicated orthopedic trauma OR and team available has benefits. First is the flexibility of the trauma cases allocated for operations. Second is the availability of a team of designated OR nurses for trauma care and fixation. This helps to shorten the operating time and the transit time between cases. Third is the availability of the anesthetists prepared for geriatric patients with trauma and patients approaching extreme age. Finally is the team of the experienced trauma surgeons. Their common goal is to help these patients safely and efficiently manage their hip fractures with the appropriate implants of prosthesis.[13]

POSTOPERATIVE CARE

Postoperative care starts in the postanesthesia area. Oral nutrition should be started as soon as a patient is awake and can tolerate and is advanced as able when on the nursing unit. Upon returning to the nursing unit, regular postoperative care guidelines are followed, along with treatment of pain. A nutrition consult and assessment may be initiated to help address common postoperative complications. Poor nutrition, dehydration, and constipation are common.[14] Patients may start mobility by sitting up at the edge of the bed with nursing or physical therapy.

POSTOPERATIVE PAIN

Pain, especially acute postoperative pain, tends to be undertreated in older patients. Poorly controlled postoperative pain in older people has been shown to be associated postoperatively with deterioration of mental status, especially delirium. On the other hand, older patients have been shown to have increased analgesic sensitivity to opioids and nonsteroidal anti-inflammatory drugs. To provide effective postoperative pain control, a scheduled pain protocol of a short-acting weak opioid in combination with nonopioid analgesic has been found beneficial in some hip fracture programs.[15]

EARLY MOBILIZATION

Early mobilization and return to preinjury level of function is the primary goal during recovery from hip fracture. Nursing can play an active role in starting to educate patients about mobilization and also by initiation of activity. Careful assessment of preinjury function and living situation must be evaluated. Goals postoperatively need to be patient-specific and attainable. Sitting up at the edge of the bed, standing, and even starting ambulation are the responsibility of nursing and therapy staff.

Mobilization is defined as any weight-bearing activity, such as standing at the bedside, transfer from bed to chair, or walking. Proponents of early mobilization argue that longer waits affect recovery through loss of muscle strength at a rate of 5% per day of bed rest. Longer waits also are associated with the occurrence of pneumonia and delirium after hip fracture surgery.[14]

Studies have identified that barriers to mobilization after hip fracture surgery include fear, lack of confidence, expectations, beliefs about the benefits and risks of activity, depression, lack of motivation, fatigue, and pain. Studies have shown patients cited fatigue and pain as the most frequent reasons for not achieving independent basic mobility or not completing their planned rehabilitation during the first 3 postoperative days. Therefore, it is essential to coordinate adequate pain management and plans for the day prior to mobilization.[14]

Mobility summary of best practice[14]

- A patient loses 5% muscle strength for every day spent in bed.
- Patients should mobilize within 24 hours of hip fracture surgery.
- Patients should mobilize at least once a day during their hospital stay.
- Mobilization is the responsibility of the entire multidisciplinary team.
- Nurses who claim responsibility for mobilizing patients as part of their professional domain lessen the risk for functional decline.

CASE MANAGEMENT

The entire multidisciplinary team coordinates the plan of care for the hip fracture patient. As discussed previously, best practice is to initiate case management upon admission. Case management is a continual, active participant in the hip fracture program. Daily rounding with other team members, patients, and patients' families ensures communication is continuous during transitions of care and handoffs. Their work is essential, as coordination of care to the rehabilitation setting remain seamless.

Sharing information related to patients' preadmission levels of function, both physical and cognitive, is critical. Access to basic information ensures a plan of care that reflects realistic goals, promotes positive clinical outcomes, and increases the quality of care.[14]

Care for the hip fracture patient can be complex with lots of moving parts. **Box 2** displays a checklist of important care elements throughout the treatment course of patients with hip fracture.

NURSING INNOVATIONS

Nursing innovations are focused on the development and coordination of a hip fracture program. This program is centered around a clinical pathway influenced by the entire multidisciplinary team. Besides basic nursing care, focus is placed on communication of multidisciplinary team members amongst themselves and to the patients and their families.

Examples of innovations in this setting include

- Whiteboard communication tool updated and utilized by all disciplines
  - Staff names
  - Goal for the day
  - Therapy times
  - Next pain medication time
  - Discharge date and destination
  - Family name and contact information
- Daily transition rounding to include patient, family, and disciplines
- Discharge planning to start on admission
- Patient education in the form of a visual tool or map focusing on mobilization and discharge

EDUCATION

Much of the nursing role involves patient education. Education focus is placed on prevention of a secondary fracture and the prevention of falls.

Because falling is the main risk factor for fractures and other injuries in elderly people and because many of the risk factors for falls and serious injuries caused by falls are similar and correctable, fall prevention is essential in the planning of effective injury prevention.[16]

Box 2

Checklist of important care elements throughout treatment course of patients with hip fracture

Preoperative and perioperative care
  Surgical team (with support of geriatric consultant, medical consultant, and primary care physician)
    ☐ Consideration of operative versus nonoperative management
  Emergency and surgical team (with support of geriatric and medical consultants)
    ☐ Adequate pain control: femoral nerve block, scheduled pain regimen, and as-needed pain regimen
    ☐ Correction of medical abnormalities prior to surgery
    ☐ Timing of surgery: early surgery but treat medical problems first
  Surgical team and anesthesia
    ☐ Regional versus general anesthesia
  Surgical team and nursing
    ☐ Prophylaxis against venous thromboembolism
    ☐ Perioperative antibiotic prophylaxis
    ☐ Pressure ulcer prevention using pressure-redistributing support surfaces, and heel elevation device

Inpatient postoperative care
  Inpatient primary team (with support of geriatric and medical consultants)
    ☐ Adequate pain control: scheduled pain regimen and preemptive pain medications
    ☐ Delirium prevention: structured protocols
    ☐ Anemia management
    ☐ Oxygen support
    ☐ Multidisciplinary inpatient care
  Rehabilitation services
    ☐ Early ambulation
  Nutrition and primary team
    ☐ Consideration for nutrition support, particularly for patients with malnutrition
  Nursing
    ☐ Urinary catheter management
    ☐ Pressure ulcer prevention
    Discharging team
    ☐ Transitions management

Rehabilitation postdischarge care
  Rehabilitation services
    ☐ Rehabilitation exercises in facilities, home, and outpatient settings
    Primary care clinicians and surgical team
    ☐ Secondary fracture prevention: bisphosphonates and fall prevention
    ☐ Monitor recovery of function
    ☐ Pain monitoring
  Primary care
    ☐ Depression monitoring and treatment
    ☐ Consideration for other modalities of care, for example, palliative care
    ☐ Communication: review trajectory of recovery and care giver expectations

---

It is beneficial to mention that a substantial amount of research and implementation has been done on the use and benefits of fracture liaison service (FLS) prevention programs. These programs provide treatment of osteoporosis and follow-up on the prevention of future fractures.

Lifestyle changes may contribute to the decrease in hip fracture incidence, with attention focused on calcium and vitamin D supplementation, avoidance of smoking, regular weight-bearing exercise, an awareness of falls, and limiting alcohol intake.[17]

OUTCOMES

Hip fracture has a prolonged treatment course with potentially devastating consequences. A patient's overall status and goals should be used to tailor care and optimize patient outcomes. Patients with hip fracture require care that integrates surgical, geriatric, rehabilitative, and psychosocial principles throughout its course. This condition also requires physicians to anticipate problems that may arise during recovery, whether the complications are from hip fracture and immobility, exacerbations of chronic diseases, or problems with social and psychological support. It takes a team of dedicated professionals working together seamlessly to deliver care appropriate for patient goals and to maximize recovery.[18]

Geriatric hip fractures used to be less attended in the past because they were considered less urgent compared with the younger patients. These fractures also traditionally were considered simple fractures to treat. This traditional approach, however, has changed rapidly in the past decade. More and more evidence has shown that osteoporotic fractures should be managed with aggressive medical and surgical support, which achieves excellent results with good clinical outcomes.[11]

SUMMARY

Hip fracture in the elderly patients is a frequent injury and serious cause of morbidity and mortality. A multidisciplinary team approach is the best way to manage this patient population to achieve the best possible outcome while attempting to return patients with hip fractures to their previous level of function. Timely surgical intervention to allow patients early mobilization decreases the risk of potential complications in the perioperative period. Patient education and close follow-up are necessary to ensure compliance with prevention of hip fractures.[9]

DISCLOSURE

The author has no financial interests, affiliations, or conflicts of interest that relate to the publication of this material.

REFERENCES

1. Management of geriatric hip fracture – care process model – Intermountain Healthcare. Available at: https://intermountainhealthcare.org/ext/Dcmnt?ncid=529346331. Accessed March 30, 2019.
2. Maggi S, Veronese N. Epidemiology and social costs of hip fracture. Injury 2018;49(8):1458–60. Available at: www.clinicalkey.com. Accessed March 30, 2019.
3. Diseases & conditions hip fractures. 2009. Available at: http://orthinfo.aaos.org/en/diseases–conditions/hip-fractures. Accessed March 19, 2019.
4. International Osteoporosis Foundation – epidemiology. 2017. Available at: http://www.iodbonehealth.org/epidemiology. Accessed February 7, 2019.
5. Hip Fracture Health Encyclopedia – University of Rochester Medical Center. Available at: https://www.urmc.rochester.edu/encyclopedia/content.aspx?ContentTypeID=85&contentID=P08957. Accessed March 30, 2019.
6. Broussard I. A clinical pathway for geriatric hip fractures. AAOSNow 2018;1–6. Accessed February 15, 2019.
7. Robertson BD, Robertson TJ. Postoperative delirium after hip fracture. J Bone Joint Surg Am 2016;88(9):2060–8. Accessed March 30, 2019.
8. Duque G, Zanker J. Rapid geriatric assessment of hip fracture. Clin Geriatr Med 2017;33(3):369–82. Available at: www.clinicalkey.com. Accessed March 30, 2019.

9. Jackman J, Watson J. Hip fractures in older men. Clin Geriatr Med 2010;26: 311–29. Available at: www.clinicalkey.com. Accessed April 19, 2019.

10. Pedersen S, Borgbjerg F, Schousboe B, et al. A comprehensive hip fracture program reduces complication rates and mortality. J Am Geriatr Soc 2008;56: 1831–8. Available at: https://onlinelibrary.wiley.com/doi/pdf/10.1111/j.1532-5415.2008.01945.x. Accessed February 15. 2009.

11. Morrison R, Siu A. Hip fracture in adults: epidemiology and medical management. Available at: www.uptodate.com. Accessed May 2, 2019.

12. Beaupre L, Jones C, Sanders L, et al. Best practices for elderly hip fracture patients. J Gen Intern Med 2005;20:1019–25. Accessed March 30, 2019.

13. Fang C, Lau T, Leung F. The effectiveness of a geriatric hip fracture clinical pathway in reducing hospital and rehabilitation length of stay and improving short-term mortality rates. Geriatr Orthop Surg Rehabil 2013;4(1):3–9. Accessed February 15, 2019.

14. Meehn A, Maher A, Brent L, et al. The international collaboration of orthopaedic nursing (ICON): Best practice nursing care standards for older adults with fragility hip fracture. Int J Orthop Trauma Nurs 2019;32:3–26. Accessed May 2, 2019.

15. Milisen K, Foreman M, Abraham I, et al. A nurse-led interdisciplinary intervention program for delirium in elderly hip-fracture patients. J Am Geriatr Soc 2001;49: 523–32. Accessed March 30, 2019.

16. Jarvinen T, Kannus P, Palvanen M, et al. Prevention of falls and consequent injuries in elderly people. Lancet 2005;366:1885–93. Accessed March 30, 2019.

17. Brauer C, Coca-Perraillon M, Cutler D, et al. Incidence and mortality of hip fractures in the United States. JAMA 2009;302(14):1573–9. Accessed March 30, 2019.

18. Egol K, Hung W, Siu A, et al. Hip fracture management tailoring care for the older patient. JAMA 2012;307(20):2185–94. Accessed March 30, 2019.

A Day in the Life

Advanced Practice Nurses Providing Care to Patients with Musculoskeletal Conditions: Preparation, Role, and Impact

Michael E. Zychowicz, DNP, ANP, ONP

KEYWORDS

- Orthopedics • Nurse practitioner • Residency • Fellowship • Education • NP
- Practice

KEY POINTS

- The presence of nurse practitioners (NPs) in orthopedics is growing steadily in a range of roles and settings.
- NPs significantly contribute to improvements in care delivery, decreased length of stay, lower cost, and increased patient satisfaction.
- Many NPs learn orthopedic practice through continuing education and on the job training.

INTRODUCTION

The role of the nurse practitioner (NP) has become an integral part of health care in the United States. The role of the NP has evolved over the past several decades to meet the needs of society. It is not clear how long NPs have been practicing in orthopedics or when they started to enter this specialty. Very little exists in the literature about orthopedic NP history. Based on this author's personal experience and practice, NPs have been in orthopedic practice since at least the 1980s. Nurses, however, have engaged in orthopedics since the late 1800s in the United Kingdom.

NPs practice in nearly every specialty and subspecialty in health care. This article provides general and orthopedic-specific information about NP education and certification. This article also describes the role, settings, and impact of the orthopedic NP on health care delivery.

HISTORIC REVIEW OF THE NURSE PRACTITIONER ROLE

The 1960s provided the backdrop for the development of an educational innovation that would change the face of health care. The birth of the NP profession happened

Orthopedic NP Specialty, Duke University School of Nursing, 307 Trent Drive, Durham, NC 27710, USA
E-mail address: Michael.Zychowicz@duke.edu

Nurs Clin N Am 55 (2020) 163–174
https://doi.org/10.1016/j.cnur.2020.02.001
0029-6465/20/© 2020 Elsevier Inc. All rights reserved.

in 1965 through a partnership between Dr Loretta Ford and Dr Henry Silver.[1] NPs have been providing high-quality care in the United States for more than 50 years.

Dr Ford, a public health nurse and faculty member at University of Colorado School of Nursing, collaborated with Dr Silver, a pediatrician, toward creating the educational foundation of an advanced role for public health nurses. Dr Ford saw a need and opportunity for public health nurses with advanced training to meet the health care needs of children.[1] Through the cooperative work of Drs Ford and Silver, the first certificate program for NPs was started at University of Colorado in 1965. A physician shortage and movement of physicians to more specialized roles helped to move the early advanced nursing role forward.[2]

Although the NP profession is relatively young, there has been tremendous growth in this role over the past 50 years. According to the American Association of Nurse Practitioners (AANP), more than 270,000 NPs are prepared for clinical practice.[3]

The profession has incrementally shifted from primary care roots toward specialty practice. Although nearly 90% of NPs indicate they are educationally prepared and board certified in a primary care role, only 40% indicate primary care as their clinical focus area.[3] With a shift away from primary care, an increasing number of NPs are finding a role in a variety of specialty practice areas including orthopedic practice.

THE FUTURE OF NURSING

To better understand the role of nursing in the ever-changing and more complex health care delivery system, the Institute of Medicine (IOM) and Robert Wood Johnson Foundation conducted a 2-year study to clarify what nursing's future role should be. In the report *The Future of Nursing: Leading Change; Advancing Health* (2010), 8 recommendations are offered to transform nursing practice, education, and leadership and meet the current and future needs of the US health care system.[4]

Although these recommendations broadly apply across the profession of nursing, some recommendations can be translated to impact orthopedic NP practice. One recommendation is to "implement nurse residency programs." This recommendation states that NPs should be supported in completion of a "transition-to-practice program (nurse residency) after they have completed a prelicensure or advanced practice degree program or when they are transitioning into new clinical practice areas."[4] One difficulty in widely developing NP residencies is the funding source to support these programs. Another recommendation that affects education and practice for orthopedic NPs is to "ensure that nurses engage in lifelong learning." Through continuing education, orthopedic NPs can obtain and maintain competence in orthopedic patient care, cutting edge therapies, and clinical skills.[4]

EDUCATION AND TRAINING

Over the 50 years of the NP profession, educational preparation for practice has evolved to meet the changing practice landscape. Initial NP education, as developed by Dr Loretta Ford, prepared nurses to become NPs with certificate training. NP education evolved to the master's degree as a minimum requirement for entry to practice. More than 80% of NPs now hold a master's degree and nearly 18% hold a doctorate degree.[3]

The NP profession has flirted with movement to DNP education as the minimum standard for entry to practice. In 2004, the American Association of Colleges of Nursing recommended moving to the DNP for entry to NP practice by 2015.[5] More recently, The National Organization of Nurse Practitioner Faculties released a 2018 position statement advocating for the requirement of the DNP for entry to NP practice by 2025.[6]

GENERAL NURSE PRACTITIONER EDUCATION

The Essentials of Master's Education in Nursing, Criteria for Evaluation of Nurse Practitioner Programs, and the *Consensus Model for APRN Regulation: Licensure, Accreditation, Certification & Education* provide foundational guidance for NP educational framework and criteria for accreditation of NP programs.[7–9] During their education, NPs engage in core master's level nursing content. They then focus on graduate courses often referred to as the "3-Ps": pathophysiology, physical assessment, and pharmacology. They then spend time on NP role courses followed by clinical management didactic and clinical practice courses focusing on the population of patients (ie, pediatric primary care) for whom they will provide care.[9]

NURSE PRACTITIONER MUSCULOSKELETAL EDUCATION

In the United States, approximately 1 in 3 people is affected by a musculoskeletal condition. Unfortunately, for most NPs, the exposure they have to orthopedic content within their graduate nursing programs is minimal. Although we have an aging population in the United States with an increasing need for musculoskeletal care, NPs receive little formal education on musculoskeletal topics.[10,11]

According to a 2016 study by Benham and Geier,[11] most NPs had fewer than 10 hours of orthopedic content during their entire graduate programs. Benham and Geier[11] also found NPs generally have lower confidence and knowledge in caring for patients with musculoskeletal conditions as compared with conditions affecting other body systems. Knowing that musculoskeletal conditions are common among patients across many settings, one could argue that the amount of musculoskeletal education NPs receive does not set a solid foundation for NPs in general practice. One could also argue the small exposure to musculoskeletal content in a typical NP program does not prepare those NPs who are interested in entering orthopedic practice.

ORTHOPEDIC NURSE PRACTITIONER WORKFORCE

Of the 270,000 NPs prepared for practice in the United States, only 1.5%, or approximately 4000, NPs describe orthopedics as their primary clinical focus.[12] This is a small percentage of the total number of NPs practicing in the United States. Of NPs with an orthopedic focus, 51% practice in private practices, 22% practice in hospital outpatient clinics, and 10% practice in hospital-based inpatient units.[12] A 2016 survey at an American Orthopedic Association (AOA) symposium, however, demonstrated that more than 75% of orthopedic surgeons who responded to the survey have an NP and/or physician's assistant (PA) on their surgical team.[10]

There is a clear need for more NPs, with relevant educational preparation, to enter the orthopedic workforce. An expanded orthopedic workforce is necessary when we consider the number of US adults older than 65 is expected to grow to at least 70 million people. This growing population will contribute to the demand for orthopedic care in the United States, which is estimated to grow by at least 50% by 2030. Compounding this increased need is a sluggish growth in the number of orthopedic surgery residents and an inability for the number of general orthopedic surgeons being trained to keep up with the number of retiring surgeons.[10,13]

A profile of the orthopedic NP workforce can be derived from a 2016 survey of nurses and nurse practitioners practicing in orthopedics. This survey was performed as a component of a role delineation study by the Orthopedic Nurses Certification Board (ONCB). In general, NPs who currently practice in orthopedics have been doing so for an average of 20 years. Most of the NPs reported they practice full time and primarily take care of an adult patient population.[14]

The 3 most common musculoskeletal conditions taken care of by orthopedic NPs, reported in the ONCB survey, include degenerative disorders, orthopedic trauma, and sport injuries. Degree preparation for orthopedic NPs mirrors that of the general NP population. Eighty-three percent of orthopedic NPs hold a master's degree and 13% hold a doctorate degree. Interestingly, approximately 4% of orthopedic NPs hold less than a master's degree in nursing.[14]

ON THE JOB TRAINING

Few formal educational programs exist to prepare orthopedic NPs for practice. Most orthopedic NPs have little or no formal advanced practice education in orthopedic care beyond their primary NP program. Most engage in "on the job" training, frequently through an apprenticeship model with an orthopedic surgeon.

Many orthopedic NPs have some foundational experience as a registered nurse in an orthopedic setting. Orthopedic nursing experience does not necessarily prepare the nurse for the greater complexity of the advanced practice role in orthopedics. The 2016 AOA surgeon survey noted previously, revealed 63% of the surgeons stated it took more than 6 months of "on the job training" until the NP or PA in their practice was where they had envisioned their performance should be.[10]

ORTHOPEDIC CONTINUING EDUCATION

Several options exist for continuing education for NPs. First, the National Association of Orthopedic Nurses (NAON) hosts an annual congress providing orthopedic-specific continuing Nursing education (CNE). The annual congress highlights an educational track for NPs and clinical nurse specialists. Other activities for NPs that are offered through NAON include live education classes, online education, and webinars.[15]

Another option for orthopedic NP continuing medical education (CME) is through the American Academy of Orthopedic Surgeons (AAOS). This organization holds an annual conference with CME. The AAOS holds a parallel track to the surgeon track for nursing and allied health professionals at the annual meeting.[16] Just as with NAON, AAOS offers a variety of CME courses and online webinars. The American College of Sports Medicine, AOA, and the Pediatric Orthopedic Society of North America all have educational offerings available for orthopedic NPs. As with other professional organizations, these organizations hold an annual educational conference in addition to online education available to members.[17–19]

Although the AANP is a generalist organization broadly representing all the NP profession, the organization has developed specialty conferences focusing on musculoskeletal care and has embedded a specialty orthopedic track within the annual conference.[20]

Last, orthopedic NPs who practice at an academic medical center may have access to onsite orthopedic CME. Orthopedic NPs can participate in the structured educational activities, such as grand rounds or case conferences, that are delivered as a part of orthopedic surgeon residency programs.

MUSCULOSKELETAL SPECIALTY EDUCATION

NP education, under the *Consensus Model for APRN Regulation*, provides guidance for embedding specialty practice curriculum for NPs within graduate programs.[9] Specialty practice education would be additive to the broad education NPs receive preparing them for their role and population. The *Consensus Model* is very clear that preparation in a specialty area of practice is not a requirement for advanced practice registered nurse (APRN) practice in that specialty area. For those who engage in additional clinical specialty education, their scope of practice does not expand. However, they do have additional focused specialty education to use within the scope of practice for their population focus.[9]

An Internet search reveals only one formal orthopedic NP specialty training program in the United States embedded in a graduate NP program. This orthopedic NP specialty program, located at Duke University School of Nursing, was founded in 2011 with funding from a Health Resources and Services Administration Advanced Nursing Education Grant.[21] Although this is currently the only program in existence, it is not the first of its kind. For several years, similar programs existed at both The University of Massachusetts Lowell School of Nursing and Rush University School of Nursing.

The program was developed to provide structured didactic and clinical education for NPs who are interested in developing a foundation of knowledge for orthopedic NP practice. Through the formal education of orthopedic NPs, the program can reduce the number of NPs who need to engage in "on the job" training. Through educating orthopedic NPs, the program may make an impact on access to care for people with orthopedic conditions.[21]

Two foundational documents from NAON were used in the development of the program: (1) *Scope and Standards of Orthopedic Nursing Practice* and (2) *Advanced Practice Resources: Graduate Curriculum, Role Descriptions, Preceptor Guidelines.*[22,23] The curriculum for this program includes 2 didactic courses, skills laboratory sessions, and a preceptored clinical rotation in orthopedics.

RESIDENCIES AND FELLOWSHIPS

Some disagreement exists around what title to use, residency or fellowship, when describing postgraduate training programs for NPs. For the purposes of this article, the term residency is used to refer to any formal postgraduate training program for NPs.[24]

One of earliest residencies, if not the first in the United States, was developed by Dr Tom Bush in 2006 at the University of North Carolina at Chapel Hill (UNC-CH). His orthopedic residency for NPs was pioneering work for those to follow. The earliest primary care NP residency is believed to have been developed in 2007 by Dr Margaret Flinter at the Community Health Center, Inc of Middletown, Connecticut.[25]

In the 2011 IOM's *Future of Nursing Report*, one key recommendation states," State boards of nursing, accrediting bodies, the federal government, and health care organizations should take actions to support nurses' completion of a transition-to-practice program (nurse residency) after they have completed a prelicensure or advanced practice degree program or when they are transitioning into new clinical practice areas."[4]

Following the IOM recommendation, NP residencies have been incrementally growing in number. According to the Association of Post-Graduate APRN Programs, more than 75 US health care organizations offer more than 115 individual NP residency training programs in a variety of specialties.[26]

Today, more than 115 residencies exist, however only 3 orthopedic NP residencies are available in the United States. The orthopedic NP residency at UNC-CH is a transition-to-practice residency that has been delivered for more than a decade. The learners are folded into activities, such as the grand rounds and lectures, with the orthopedic surgery resident training program. The NP residents initially work closely with a surgeon but have progressively greater autonomy as they advance along their training program. The residents engage in a wide variety of clinical experiences including taking calls for the orthopedic service.[27]

Two additional residency programs are located at the Carillion Clinic in Virginia and at the Medical College of Wisconsin. Both programs offer a 1-year combined PA and NP training program. They have structured orthopedic clinical and didactic education through an interprofessional program along with their orthopedic surgeon residency program. Each program delivers a variety of core curriculum topic areas preparing the residents for practice.[28,29]

CERTIFICATION

Nurses and NPs have the option of obtaining board certification through the ONCB. The ONCB began in 1986 with a mission toward improving "musculoskeletal health by providing nurses with certifications that promote professional development and advance the practice of orthopedic nursing."[30] The Orthopedic Nurse–Certified (ONC) certification began in 1988 as a mechanism to recognize clinical expertise and foundational knowledge of nurses practicing in orthopedic settings.

The Orthopedic Clinical Nurse Specialist–Certified (OCNS-C) and the Orthopedic Nurse Practitioner–Certified (ONP-C) certifications became available through ONCB in 2006. Unfortunately, the OCNS-C certification was discontinued in 2014. ONCB remains the only option for board certification for orthopedic nurses and NPs. More than 10,000 nurses in the United States, Hong Kong, and Canada have become ONC-certified, whereas only 160 NPs have earned the ONP-C certification.[14]

PRACTICE MODELS

Three general clinical practice models are used for incorporating NPs into orthopedic practice. One model involves the surgeon and the NP collaborating closely to see all patients together. In this model, the NP may initially evaluate the patient and gather diagnostic imaging or other patient data. The surgeon would then join the NP and the patient to evaluate the findings and finalize a treatment plan. The NP would then spend time with the patient delivering any necessary education and planning.[31–33]

Some believe this physician extender model increases the volume of patients who can be seen by a physician through reducing the amount of time a physician needs to spend with each patient.[31] This model is believed to be less satisfying for NPs because of less practice autonomy, along with underutilization of the NPs' skill set.[32]

A second model described in the literature involves the NP integrated in a practice in a highly independent fashion. This model takes advantage of the NPs' full scope of practice in the clinical setting contributing to patient continuity of care.[31] The NP would independently take care of new and established patients that fall within the scope of practice and skill set for the NP. The NP would also refer patients to a surgeon in the practice if the patient requires, or would benefit from, surgical intervention. Patients who fall outside of the NP's scope of practice or skill set would also be referred to the surgeon for evaluation and management.[32,33] This model is understood to decrease patient wait time through increasing access to care.[32]

The third model by which NPs practice in orthopedics involves a team approach. In this model, the NP would be part of a care delivery team that distributes the patient load across the team members. These teams are frequently composed of interdisciplinary health care providers and are generally employed in an acute setting. The model potentially has a decreased continuity of care for those patients being cared for by the team.[31,32]

Many practices will use a variation of one of the preceding models or a combination of more than one of the models.[33] In addition, practices will either have the NP partner in a 1:1 fashion with a single surgeon or partner with a group of surgeons.[31,32]

PRACTICE SETTINGS AND IMPACT

Orthopedic NPs practice in several different settings assuming a variety of roles. Broadly, NPs contribute to health care though lowering health care costs and increasing access to high-quality care. Little has been captured in the literature specifically describing orthopedic NP impact on care for orthopedic patients.

OUTPATIENT CLINIC

The role of the orthopedic NP in the outpatient setting frequently revolves around evaluating and managing the care of new or established patients. This may be conducted through using any of the practice models described previously. In the outpatient orthopedic setting, NPs may conduct preoperative assessments and educate patients as well as deliver postoperative patient care. Tasks can include joint or soft tissue injections, fracture management, treatment of sprains and strains, and wound management. NPs will order and interpret diagnostic tests and imaging studies. These outpatient NPs may also have an additional role in assisting at surgery, rounding on hospitalized patients, or being on-call.[32,33]

In a 2014 article, Horn and colleagues[34] provide a retrospective assessment of the implementation of an NP into their practice. This model provided a 1:1 paired NP with a surgeon at a pediatric trauma hospital orthopedic clinic. The NP in this study practiced collaboratively with the surgeon to evaluate and manage pediatric patients. In this model, the surgeon typically evaluated the new patients, with follow-up care going to the NP. Most patients who required fracture follow-up care also were managed by the NP.[34]

The investigators describe their physician-NP model as leading to increased access to care through an increased volume of patients seen in the practice. Not only was there an increase in overall patient volume with this model, the volume of surgical cases increased for the service as well. Last, following the implementation of a 1:1 paired physician-NP model, patient satisfaction improved.[34]

In a 2010 study of an NP-managed outpatient osteoporosis program in California, Green and Dell[35] described the impact of their model on osteoporosis care and the potential impact on osteoporosis-related hip fractures. The NP in this program worked with an interdisciplinary team to identify patients who are at risk for, or have, osteoporosis and/or insufficiency fractures. The NP worked with the patients to educate them about the disease and to manage the care for this population of patients.[35]

Over a 5-year period of the NP-led osteoporosis program, the program demonstrated a 914% increase in the number of patients obtaining a dual-energy x-ray absorptiometry scan. With this increase in screening for osteoporosis, the number of patients who were started on antiosteoporosis medication increased by more than 150%. A significant impact of this program was the reduction in projected hip fracture rate by 38% in this population of patients.[35]

EXEMPLAR

Dr Tom Bush has been providing orthopedic care as an NP at the UNC Health System for nearly 19 years. Dr Bush's initial foray into orthopedics was as a first assistant in surgery, practicing on a sports medicine and hand surgery service. In addition to assisting in the operating room (OR), Dr Bush collaborated with the surgeons to evaluate preoperative and postoperative patients in the outpatient clinic.[36]

Yearning for a more independent role and seeing a need for increasing access to orthopedic care because of a decreasing number of orthopedic providers, Dr Bush advocated to change his practice model. He eventually left his work in the OR to develop an outpatient primary care musculoskeletal clinic where he independently managed his own panel of patients.[36]

As a Family NP, Dr Bush developed a niche focus of screening pediatric patients who have lower extremity malalignment conditions. Many of these pediatric malalignment conditions do not require surgery. He is able to effectively evaluate these patients and refer the small number who require surgical intervention to the appropriate surgical consultation. Dr Bush now practices in an outpatient orthopedic urgent care setting where he provides episodic care for patients who have acute nonsurgical injuries. He also contributes to the education of the family medicine physician residents who rotate through his musculoskeletal clinic.[36]

PREOPERATIVE SETTING

Examination and preoperative evaluation of a patient is essential for the assessment of perioperative risk. Orthopedic NPs practicing in this role may perform preoperative assessments within a dedicated clinic setting or as a service within a surgical practice for elective surgeries. In addition, the NP can engage in this role in the emergency room (ER) before urgent or emergent orthopedic surgeries.[32]

Using accepted practice guidelines, the NP can optimize the patient medically before surgery, potentially reducing perioperative risk.[32,37,38] Dedicated preoperative clinics can have a positive effect on patient care in enhancing care coordination and improving patient satisfaction with the surgical experience. By having NPs conduct preoperative assessments at dedicated clinics for elective surgeries, instead of having the patient seek clearance through their primary care provider, a reduction in the amount of lead time to schedule a surgical procedure can be reduced.[38]

Sebach and colleagues[38] studied the impact of implementing an NP-led preoperative clinic as part of an orthopedic practice. They compared the volume of surgical cancellations before and after the implementation of their dedicated NP-led preoperative clinic. Before implementation of this model, the practice had a 7.7% surgical cancellation rate. Following implementation, the cancellation rate dropped to 0.8%, demonstrating a statistically significant relationship between implementation of this role and decreased surgical cancellations. This reduced cancellation rate translated to an increase in surgical revenue for the practice.[39]

ACUTE CARE

Orthopedic NPs who practice in the acute care or inpatient setting, typically practice in a collaborative fashion as part of a multidisciplinary team. These NPs are often responsible for rounding on postoperative patients and ordering or interpreting diagnostic tests or imaging. Acute care orthopedic NPs may assist with surgery and manage orthopedic patients that present to the ER. They will coordinate and deliver patient care, including placing or removing drains, dressing changes, wound assessments, pin care or pin removal, and placing or removing casts. These NPs also will have a central role in providing education to patients and their families and engaging in discharge planning and education.[32,39–41]

A 2012 study highlights the impact of employing an orthopedic NP team member on a Canadian hip fracture care team between 1998 through 2010. Through putting in place standardized clinical pathways and using a care coordination approach, the NP was able to significantly reduce the length of stay (LOS) for patients with hip fracture. When the role of the acute care orthopedic NP was initiated in this Canadian hospital in 1998, LOS for patients with hip fracture was 33.1 days for those between 65 and 79 years old and 39 days for those older than 80 years. There was a drop in LOS over the first 3 years of implementation to 13 days for those 65 to 79 years and 19 days for those older than 80 years. The LOS for all patients continued to decrease through 2010 to a median LOS of 6 days.[39]

A 2017 retrospective study of Australian orthopedic NP care demonstrated decreased LOS and decreased cost following the implementation of the NP role on an acute orthopedic team. This study compared data from patients before and after the implementation of the orthopedic NP role on the surgical service. In comparing patient data from 2010 and 2013, the average patient was female and 84 years of age. The data demonstrated a significant decrease in LOS for patients between 2010 and 2013 (5.3–4.4 days). An estimated per-patient cost reduction was >$1100 per patient. A correlation was found between LOS and other confounding factors. Urinary tract infection as well as cardiovascular, pulmonary, and neuropsychiatric comorbidities were correlated with greater LOS for patients in the study. Decreased time getting a patient to the OR as well as the type of surgical approach selected by the surgeon was correlated with a decreased LOS.[40]

A similar 2015 study by Hiza and colleagues[41] evaluated orthopedic patient outcomes before and after implementation of the NP role on a surgical service at a large level 1 trauma center in the United States. Following a chart review of patients between 2011 and 2013, a 1-year cohort of patients discharged before the NP joined the surgical team were compared with a group of patients discharged 1 year after the NP joined the team. There was a significant reduction in LOS, dropping from 6.02 days to 4.91 days after the NP joined the surgical team.[41]

The investigators evaluated subgroups of patients discharged from the trauma service to find a significant reduction in LOS for patients discharged to rehabilitation, discharged with antibiotics and wound vacuum assisted closure (VAC) devices, and those older than 60 years. Although not statistically significant, length of time for a patient to get to the OR after admission through the ER was reduced from 1.48 days to 1.31 days. The investigators estimated the indirect cost savings with the implementation of the NP role on this orthopedic surgical service is greater than $1,000,000.[41]

EXEMPLAR

Mrs Maggie Harding is an NP who practices on the inpatient orthopedic surgery unit at the Duke University Health System. In her role, she manages all the postoperative care and medical management for the orthopedic surgery patients on the unit. She initially realized she enjoyed orthopedic care while she was practicing as a nurse in the post-anesthesia care setting.[42]

A typical day for her includes managing wound care, pin care, wound VACs, immobilization devices, and traction. She evaluates and clears postoperative patient radiographs with the orthopedic team. She also has a big role in discharge planning and patient education, coordinating care with a case manager, and ensuring all needed prescriptions and referrals are in place for when the patients are discharged.[42]

During more than 5 years of orthopedic NP practice, Mrs Harding has taken advantage of the wealth of educational opportunities available to her at an academic medical center. She has become more confident and independent in her practice over time and has now added a surgical assisting component to her role. In addition to significantly impacting patient care, she believes the role of the unit-based orthopedic NP in the acute care setting is a benefit for the nurses on the unit. As an NP, she is able to spend time teaching the nurses on the unit. She is also a readily available provider for nurses to go to with patient care issues or questions, eliminating the need for nurses to track down a resident or attending.[42]

SUMMARY

It is well documented that nurses have contributed to the practice of orthopedics since the Victorian age. Unfortunately, the early history of NP engagement in orthopedic care is somewhat unknown.

Despite a growing number of NPs practicing in orthopedic settings, as well as the large volume of musculoskeletal complaints addressed in nonorthopedic settings, it remains surprising that more time is not dedicated to the formal education of NPs around orthopedic patient care topics. As a profession, more formal educational opportunities about orthopedic topics is needed so our clinicians do not have to rely on informal "on the job" training. We have an ethical obligation to society to ensure our clinicians are well trained for the practice they are to enter.

Even with many NPs relying on informal "on the job" education and continuing education, the NPs of today significantly contribute to the care or orthopedic patients in many roles and a variety of settings. The high-quality care delivered by NPs in orthopedic settings has become an integral part of the larger orthopedic care delivery team and should continue to grow and expand into the future.

DISCLOSURE

The authors have nothing to disclose.

REFERENCE

1. Ford LC. Reflections on 50 years of change. J Am Assoc Nurse Pract 2015;27(6): 294–5.
2. Ralston B, Collier TH. The NP: celebrating 50 years. Am J Nurs 2015; 115(10):54–7.
3. All about NPs. American Association of Nurse Practitioners. Available at: https://www.aanp.org/about/all-about-nps. Accessed June 2, 2019.
4. Committee on The Robert Wood Johnson Foundation Initiative. Future of nursing - leading change, advancing health. Washington, DC: National Academies Press; 2010.
5. AACN Position Statement on the Practice Doctorate in Nursing. American Association of Colleges of Nursing. Available at: https://www.aacnnursing.org/DNP/Position-Statement. Accessed June 1, 2019.
6. The Doctor of Nursing Practice Degree: Entry to Nurse Practitioner Practice by 2025. National Organization of Nurse Practitioner Faculties. Available at: https://cdn.ymaws.com/www.nonpf.org/resource/resmgr/dnp/v3_05.2018_NONPF_DNP_Stateme.pdf. Accessed June 1, 2019.
7. American Association of Colleges of Nursing. The essentials of masters education in nursing. Washington, DC: American Association of Colleges of Nursing; 2011.
8. National Task Force on Quality Nurse Practitioner Education. 2016 criteria for evaluation of nurse practitioner programs. 5th edition. Washington, DC: NONPF; 2016.

9. APRN Consensus Work Group & the National Council of State Boards of Nursing APRN Advisory Committee. Consensus model for APRN regulation: licensure, accreditation, certification & education. Chicago (IL): National Council of State Boards of Nursing; 2008.

10. Day CS, Bodon SD, Knott PT, et al. Musculoskeletal workforce needs: are physician assistants and nurse practitioners the solution? J Bone Joint Surg Am 2016; 98(e46):1–6.

11. Benham AJ, Geier KA. How well are nurse practitioners prepared to treat common musculoskeletal conditions? Orthop Nurs 2016;35(5):325–9.

12. American Association of Nurse Practitioners. 2018 National Sample Survey of Nurse Practitioners. Custom data analysis of NPs requested May 21, 2019.

13. Instone SL, Palmer DM. Bringing the institute of medicine's report to life: developing a doctor of nursing practice orthopedic residency. J Nurs Educ 2013; 52(2):116–9.

14. Roberts D, Pirri K, Hanes M. Keeping up with current orthopaedic nursing practice: results of the ONCB 2016 role delineation study. Orthop Nurs 2019;38(4): 234–41.

15. Education. NAON. Available at: http://www.orthonurse.org/page/education. Accessed June 1, 2019.

16. Education. Available at: https://www.aaos.org/education/. Accessed June 1, 2019.

17. Upcoming Meetings & Conferences. ACSM Events Meetings Conferences. Available at: https://www.acsm.org/attend-connect/events-and-conferences. Accessed June 1, 2019.

18. Advanced Solutions International, Inc. AOA Meetings & Education. Meetings and Education Overview. Available at: https://www.aoassn.org/aoaimis/AOANEW/Meetings___and___Education/AOANEW/Meetings___and___Education/Meetings___and___Education___Overview.aspx?hkey=e74991e0-cef6-4955-983b-41d47ded94d8. Accessed June 2, 2019.

19. POSNA Meetings. POSNA. Available at: https://posna.org/Physician-Education. Accessed June 2, 2019.

20. Education. American Association of Nurse Practitioners. Available at: https://www.aanp.org/education. Accessed June 1, 2019.

21. Orthopedics Specialty. Duke University School of Nursing. 2019. Available at: https://nursing.duke.edu/academic-programs/msn-master-science-nursing/orthopedics-specialty. Accessed May 30, 2019.

22. Harvey CV, David J, Eckhouse DR, et al. The National Association of Orthopaedic Nurses (NAON) scope and standards of orthopaedic nursing practice. Orthop Nurs 2013;32(3):139–52.

23. Bianchi C, Gates SJ, Green J, et al. National association of orthopedic nurses advanced practice resources: graduate curriculum, role descriptions, preceptor guidelines. 2nd edition. Pitman (PA): Jannetti; 2002.

24. Nicely KLW, Fairman J. Postgraduate nurse practitioner residency programs: supporting transition to practice. Acad Med 2015;90(6):707–9.

25. Training to Complexity. Training for the Future. Nurse Practitioner Residency Training Program. Available at: https://www.npresidency.com/. Accessed May 30, 2019.

26. Association of Post Graduate APRN Programs | ENP Network. Available at: https://apgap.enpnetwork.com/. Accessed May 30, 2019.

27. UNC Orthopaedic NP Fellowship. Association of Post Graduate APRN Programs | ENP Network. Available at: https://apgap.enpnetwork.com/nurse-practitioner-news/140511-unc-orthopaedic-np-fellowship. Accessed June 1, 2019.
28. Orthopaedics Surgery ACP Fellowship. Available at: https://www.carilionclinic.org/orthopaedics/fellowship-acp. Accessed May 30, 2019.
29. MCW Advanced Practice Providers. Medical College of Wisconsin. Available at: https://www.mcw.edu/departments/mcw-advanced-practice-providers/app-fellowship-programs/app-orthopaedic-fellowship. Accessed May 30, 2019.
30. ONP-C® Certification. Orthopaedic Nurses Certification Board. Available at: https://www.oncb.org/certifications/onp-c-certification/. Accessed May 30, 2019.
31. Dower C, Christian S. Physician assistants and nurse practitioners in specialty care: six practices make it work. San Francisco (CA): Center for the Health Professions, University of California; 2009.
32. Spence BG, Ricci J, McCuaig F. Nurse practitioners in orthopaedic surgical settings: a review of the literature. Orthop Nurs 2019;38(1):17–24.
33. Ward WT, Eberson CP, Otis SA, et al. Pediatric orthopaedic practice management: the role of midlevel providers. J Pediatr Orthop 2008;28(8):795–8.
34. Horn P, Badowski E, Klingele K. Orthopaedic clinical care model in a pediatric orthopedic setting: outcomes of a 1:1 model-orthopaedic surgeon and nurse practitioner. Orthop Nurs 2014;33(3):142–6.
35. Green D, Dell RM. Outcomes of an osteoporosis disease-management program managed by a nurse practitioner. J Am Acad Nurse Pract 2010;22(2010):326–9.
36. Zychowicz ME. Interview with Dr. Tom Bush, NP. May 2019.
37. Johnson JP. Preoperative assessment of high-risk orthopedic surgery patients. Nurse Pract 2011;36(7):40–7.
38. Sebach AM, Rochelli LA, Reddish W, et al. Development of a nurse practitioner-managed preoperative evaluation clinic within a multispecialty orthopedic practice. J Nurse Pract 2015;11(9):869–77.
39. Forster FJ. Developing a nurse practitioner role for hip fracture care: a journey of challenges. Int J Orthop Trauma Nurs 2012;16:214–21.
40. Coventry LL, Pickles S, Sin M, et al. Impact of the orthopedic nurse practitioner role on acute hospital length of stay and cost-savings for patients with hip fracture: a retrospective cohort study. J Adv Nurs 2017;73:2652–63.
41. Hiza EA, Gottschalk MB, Umpierrez E, et al. Effect of a dedicated orthopedic advanced practice provider in a level 1 trauma center: analysis of length of stay and cost. J Orthop Trauma 2015;29(7):e225–30.
42. Zychowicz ME. Interview with Mrs. Maggie Harding, NP. May 2019.

Emerging Spine Care Trends and Innovations

Dorothy Pietrowski, MSN, ACNP, ONP-C

KEYWORDS

- Compression fracture • Herniated disc • Spine • Spinal stenosis
- Spinal rehabilitation • Spondylolisthesis • Spondylosis

KEY POINTS

- Identify common anatomic structures and functions of the spine.
- Discuss signs and symptoms of spinal disorders.
- Determine management options, including the patient clinical pathway through the continuum.
- Describe trending innovations and possible future treatment options in optimization.

INTRODUCTION

Treatment of spinal disorders continues to be one of the leading causes for office and acute care visits despite changes in treatment options and algorithms. Studies are consistent in concluding the need for preventative care in at-risk populations. Age, sex, and race are 3 factors that increase a patient's risk for developing back pain and needing emergency care.[1] Furthermore, there are increased concerns for those who are disabled, depressed, and socioeconomically disadvantaged.[2] As educators and innovators, caregivers are tasked with decoding the demographics of each individual's situation and then using available tools to improve outcomes.

Understanding the anatomy, function, and normal aging processes of the spine has been the cornerstone of treatment and research. The goal of technological advances is to continue to push the envelope, allowing patients to return to activity and achieve optimum quality of life at a faster rate. Treatment opportunities in robotics, biologics, and rehabilitation will continue to evolve into how spine patients are treated through the continuum of their given diagnosis.

SPINAL ANATOMY

At the core of the musculoskeletal system lies a vertebral column that comprises the spine; 33 vertebrae are separated into 5 regions (**Fig. 1**). The cervical, thoracic, and

Department of Orthopaedic Surgery and Rehabilitative Services, University of Chicago, 5841 South Maryland MC3079, Chicago, IL 60637, USA
E-mail address: dpietrowski@bsd.uchicago.edu

Nurs Clin N Am 55 (2020) 175–192
https://doi.org/10.1016/j.cnur.2020.02.008
0029-6465/20/© 2020 Elsevier Inc. All rights reserved.

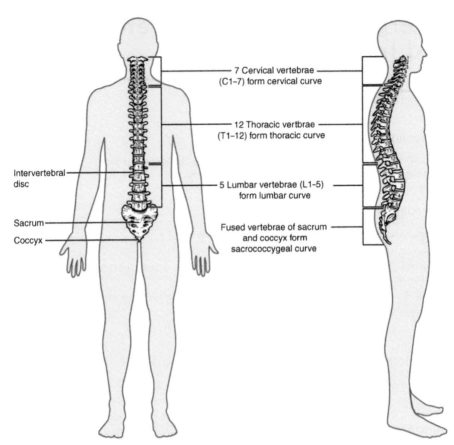

Intervertebral disc

7 Cervical vertebrae (C1–7) form cervical curve

12 Thoracic vertbrae (T1–12) form thoracic curve

5 Lumbar vertebrae (L1-5) form lumbar curve

Sacrum

Coccyx

Fused vertebrae of sacrum and coccyx form sacrococcygeal curve

Fig. 1. The spinal column. (*From* OpenStax College, Anatomy & Physiology. Connexions Web site; 2013. Retrieved from http://cnx.org/content/col11496/1.6/.)

lumbar sections are mobile and contribute to the spine's total range of motion at varying degrees. The sacrum and coccygeal areas are fused. From the top of the cervical spine to the base of the lumbar, the vertebrae get incrementally larger. The cervical and lumbar spines have a normal lordotic posture, whereas the thoracic spine is kyphotic in nature.

The cervical spine is composed of 7 vertebrae and include the atlas (C1) and the axis (C2). These 2 vertebrae account for approximately half of all the range of motion in the cervical spine when considering flexion, extension, and rotation. The thoracic spine, or midback, consists of 12 vertebrae. The motion allowed in the thoracic spine is markedly less due to the rib cage and the sternum. The 5 vertebrae of the lumbar spine support the weight of the body and as such are the largest in size.

There are anatomic structures that are common to each region of the spine, but most possess a similar body (**Fig. 2**). Behind the body are structures that encircle the neural structures of the spinal cord and nerves. These structures are the pedicles and lamina. The transverse and spinous processes function as levers and allow for attachments of muscles. The superior and inferior articular processes, or facets, allow for gliding movement between vertebral bodies and maintain stabilization. Ligaments help stabilize the spine from one vertebra to the next. The most commonly discussed

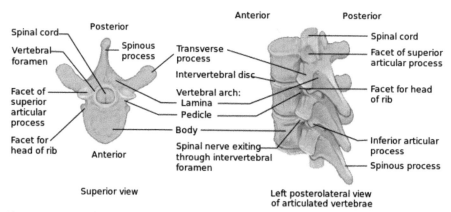

Fig. 2. Bony spinal anatomy. (*From* Jmarchn, Anatomy & Physiology. Connexions Web site; 2015. Retrieved from http://cnx.org/content/col11496/1.6/.)

are the anterior longitudinal ligament and posterior longitudinal ligament (PLL), the interspinous, and ligamentum flavum.

The intervertebral discs' primary function is to absorb stresses while allowing for mobility. There are 2 parts that compose the structure: the annulus fibrosus and the nucleus pulposus. The annulus consists of collagen fibers that are organized in concentric layers. The purpose of these layers is to provide strength and elasticity. The pulposus is soft, gelatinous, and made up of proteoglycans. With time, and as part of the normal aging process, water content is lost in the pulposus, leading to degenerative changes and loss of function. The eventual breakdown of proteoglycans reduces this hydration.[3]

All vertebrae possess a central passage, or foramen, that is most commonly called the spinal canal. It is within the canal that the spinal cord and nerves reside. The cord itself runs through the cervical and thoracic spine, terminating at or near L1. This termination is a collection of lumbar, sacral, and coccygeal nerve roots and is called the cauda equina; 31 pairs of spinal nerve roots leave the canal through the neuroforamen and innervate specific areas of the body (**Fig. 3**). Typically, it is the dermatomal pattern of a patient's symptoms that assists in diagnosis and treatment.[4]

DIAGNOSTICS

Imaging tests and nerve function testing are tools used to further understand spinal pathologies. A standard radiograph should be taken in at least 2 planes of the spine to show bony structure, so that alignment can be assessed, along with any abnormalities, such as fracture or loss of disc height. Flexion and extension views are helpful in assessing any dynamic instability between vertebral bodies after falls, accidents, and trauma.[5] Open mouth views are important in the visualization of the odontoid and for any concerning asymmetry or displacement in patients, such as those diagnosed with rheumatoid arthritis.[6] Oblique radiograph taken at a 45° angle may show fractures in the pars interarticularis, seen more commonly in adolescents.[7]

Plain radiographs do not directly show deficiencies in soft tissue structures, neuroelements, ligaments, or intervertebral discs. Magnetic resonance imaging (MRI) is considered the study of choice due to the ability to diagnose annular tears, infections, cysts, edema, myelomalacia, and degeneration through changes in signal on weighted images or enhancement.[6,8,9] The MRI allows for images to be taken in

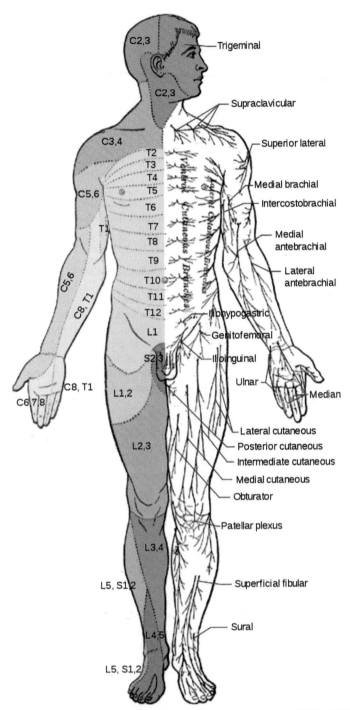

Fig. 3. Dermatomes. (*From* Häggström M, Wikimedia Commons; 2010. Retrieved from https://commons.wikimedia.org/w/index.php?curid=11803486.)

multiple planes, allowing for better visualization and clarity for a diagnosis (**Fig. 4**). Intravenous dye can be used to further augment the images from MRI to help differentiate between normal tissue, tumor, infection, or postoperative scar.[10]

Computed tomography (CT) scans are utilized for confirmation of fracture or fracture pattern. CT myelography utilizes dye to enhance the visualization of stenosis due to degeneration, disc herniation, or tumor.[11] The use of CT myelography is less than MRI due to the increased amounts of radiation in CT along with risk factors associated with the injection of dye into the spinal canal.[12] In times of trauma, a CT scan is faster to assist with diagnosis than MRI. MRI scanning of the spine may not be possible for patients with stents, clips, or pacemakers that are not compatible. In this case, CT scans or CT myelograms are the next best choice in diagnostic imaging.

Electromyography (EMG) and nerve conduction studies (NCSs) assist in differentiating diagnoses from the central and peripheral nervous systems. These tests can be helpful in diagnosing neuromuscular disorders, radiculopathy, peripheral nerve issues (ie, carpal or cubital tunnel syndromes), and immune disorders, such as Guillain-Barré. They also are useful in differentiating between a central nerve root issue versus a peripheral compression.[13]

SPINAL DISORDERS AND CLINICAL PRESENTATIONS

A leading cause for disease burden worldwide continues to be nonspecific back pain.[14] Clinical diagnosis of spinal disorders always should begin with a thorough understanding of the history and a comprehensive physical examination. Identifying common disease processes and presentations help formulate a plan that allows patients to return to activity at an accelerated rate. As educators and advocates, this knowledge also can be used in the preventative care setting to decrease the problem in these patient populations.

A strain is one of the more common diagnoses caused by acute traumatic events that can become chronic in nature if not addressed appropriately. Factors that

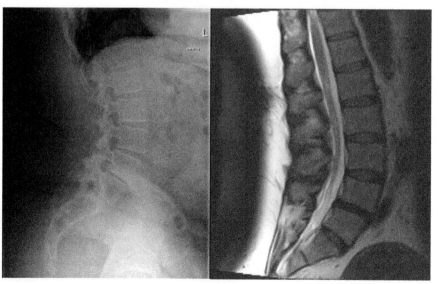

Fig. 4. Lumbar views in radiograph and MRI. (*Courtesy of* Pietrowski D, MSN ACNP ONP-C, Chicago, IL.)

increase risk of chronic symptoms are age, female sex, lower income, and multiple chronic comorbidities.[15] Patients present with muscular pain that is increased with range of motion and/or manipulation. The mechanical nature of symptoms may be due to overuse, degenerative changes, or an acute injury to the muscle, disc, or ligaments.

Degenerative Disc Disease and Disc Herniations

Degenerative disc disease is a universal term used to describe wear and tear, or arthritic changes, in the spine. Degenerative changes happen as the disc loses water content and alters the mechanical forces through that segment. Disc herniations can contribute to early disc space issues. Over time, degenerative changes to the bony structure may occur, including the endplates of the vertebral bodies and the facet joints (**Fig. 5**). Osteophytes or cysts can form, further decreasing range of motion and increasing pain.

Disc herniations are a result of the central gelatinous core of a disc progressing through a fissure or tear in the outer core or annulus. Many disc herniations can cause radicular-type symptoms in a dermatomal fashion with pain, changes in sensation, or weakness. Causes of disc herniations can be acute in nature or due to wear and tear over time. In the cervical spine, the C5-6 disc is most common to herniate, whereas in

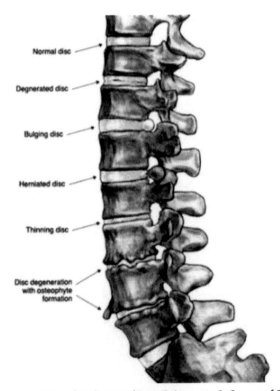

Fig. 5. Causes of degenerative disc disease. (*From* Spinasanta S. Causes of Degenerative Disc Disease. Spine Universe, Remedy Health Media, LLC. https://www.spineuniverse.com/conditions/degenerative-disc/causes-degenerative-disc-disease. Updated April 1, 2019. Feb 5, 2020. Used with Permission. © 2020 SpineUniverse.com, Remedy Health Media, LLC.)

the lumbar spine, L5-S1 is most common (**Fig. 6**). Compression testing in the neck, and straight leg testing for the lumbar spine are most sensitive for diagnosis.

Cauda equina syndrome (CES) is one of the few orthopedic emergencies that can be caused by a disc herniation or any other canal occupying lesion, such as tumor, infection, hematoma, or severe degenerative disease.[16–18] The result of compression on the spinal cord, cauda equina, or nerve roots can present as pain, loss of motor function, sensation loss, bowel and or bladder disfunction, saddle anesthesia, impotence, and back pain. Spasticity and hyperreflexia may be other indicators of CES.[19] A thorough physical examination should include documentation of motor strength, sensation to pinprick, sphincter tone, and possibly a bulbocavernosus reflex. This baseline examination is used to compare progression of symptoms based on intervention. An emergent MRI is warranted for confirmation of CES.

Spondylolysis and Spondylolisthesis

A stress fracture in the pars interarticularis is defined as a spondylolysis. This diagnosis is discovered most commonly in adolescents, particularly in those involved in sports that involve repeated hyperextension of the spine. The highest incidence is in those who participate in gymnastics/dance, football (linemen), rugby, wrestling, and martial arts.[20] The most common vertebral level involved is L5, with a prevalence of approximately 6% of the population.

Most adolescents describe back pain with range of motion, with or without a radicular component, as a nerve root can be irritated, causing leg pain or sensation changes.[20,21] Due to the competitive nature of so many sports, there can be a significant delay in diagnosis and treatment in these patients, leading to complications of nonunion, chronic pain, and spinal instability.[22] Patients complain of tenderness to palpation and with extension of the lumbar spine. They also may complain of sitting and standing intolerance for longer periods of time. Hamstrings tend to be tight in these athletes, which is a precursor to injury.[23] Plain radiographs, MRI, CT scans, and bone scans can be used to confirm whether the fracture is bilateral or unilateral.

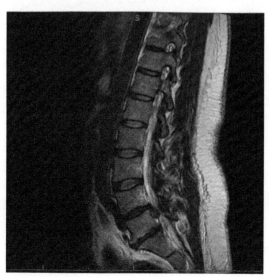

Fig. 6. Sagittal view of the lumbar spine with a disc herniation at L4-5. (*Courtesy of* Pietrowski D, MSN ACNP ONP-C, Chicago, IL.)

Translation of one vertebra over another is defined as, *spondylolisthesis*. The term is derived from the Greek root *spondylos*, which means vertebra, and *olisthesis*, which means to slip or slide. One of the concerns for a pars fracture is the development of an anterolisthesis of one vertebrae on the other, causing stenosis or narrowing of the central canal and/or neuroforamen (**Fig. 7**). The most commonly used classification system for spondylolisthesis is Wiltse-Newman, which describes 5 types or causes (**Table 1**). The Marchetti-Bartolozzi system further disseminates developmental or acquired slips and adds postsurgical or iatrogenic causes. The Myerding classification grades the severity of the slip from I to V (**Table 2**).

The most common form of spondylolisthesis is degenerative in nature and is most common in women over the age of 50 at the L4-5 level.[24] Most of the degenerative process is due to loss of water content in the intervertebral disc along with changes in the facet joint causing instability. A patient can be living with a spondylolisthesis for a long time without feeling any mechanical or neurologic effects. Many times, there is some sort of repetitive activity or trauma that can trigger symptoms.

With spondylolisthesis, the chief complaint is pain at the level of the slip with or without referral into the extremities. Patients can complain of sciatic symptoms with pain and sensation changes following a dermatomal pattern. The L5 nerve root passes centrally at the L4-5 while exiting at L5-S1. An L5 palsy can present as weakness in dorsiflexion or extensor hallucis longus on the compressed side.[25] The symptoms

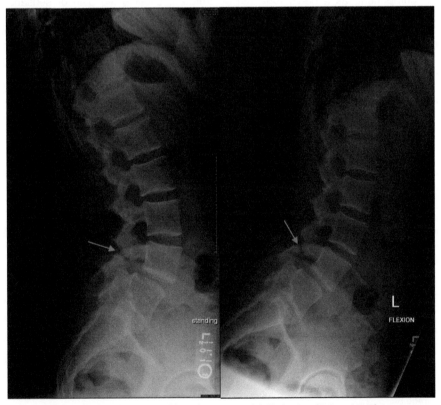

Fig. 7. Lateral radiograph of unstable isthmic spondylolisthesis of L4 on L5. The arrows are pointing at a spondylolysis. (*Courtesy of* Pietrowski D, MSN ACNP ONP-C, Chicago, IL.)

Table 1
Wiltse-Newman classification of spondylolisthesis

Type I	Congenital
Type II	Isthmic
Type III	Degenerative
Type IV	Traumatic
Type V	Neoplastic

are reproducible with ambulation and extension of the spine. Upright radiographs in neutral, flexion, and extension allow for assessment of segmental instability. MRI assesses central and neuroforaminal compression that may be contributing to the overall presentation.

Spinal Stenosis

The physical reduction in space within the spinal canal is defined as spinal stenosis. Primary stenosis is congenital in nature, presenting with a spinal canal that is more narrow than usual. Acquired stenosis also can occur in any region of the spine and is due most commonly to degenerative changes of the vertebral elements (osteoarthritis), spondylolisthesis, disc herniations, or injury. The concern with stenosis in the cervical and thoracic spine is the risk of spinal cord compression and dysfunction, such as in ossification of the posterior longitudinal ligament (OPLL), disc herniations, and traumatic dislocations (**Fig. 8**). In the lumbar spine, other differential causes include cysts, overgrowth of the facet joint, and buckling of the ligamentum flavum.

Cervical and thoracic stenosis

Patients with cervical or thoracic stenosis may have difficulty with gait and a general declining loss in function. Patients may present with symptoms of cord dysfunction (myelopathy), such as difficulty with dexterity, sensation loss, a sense of heaviness in the extremities, and muscle wasting.[26,27] Their gait also may be ataxic in nature. Associated symptoms may include bladder incontinence, imbalance, and falls. In the elderly population, they may write off these symptoms as vertigo, or a normal progression of the aging process. Progression of myelopathy can take long periods of time, with a stepwise decline and plateau in symptoms.

On examination, gait should be assessed first, including observation of a patient's gaze, because many times patients watch their feet placement due to cord dysfunction. With sudden decline in function, a patient may present in a wheelchair. A full head-to-toe assessment needs to be completed and documented for future assessments to check for progression. Inspect the patient and note any sagittal imbalance

Table 2
Myerding classification—based on percentage of slip

College	Percent Translation
Grade I	<25%
Grade II	25%–50%
Grade III	50%–75%
Grade IV	75%–100%
Grade V	Spondyloptosis

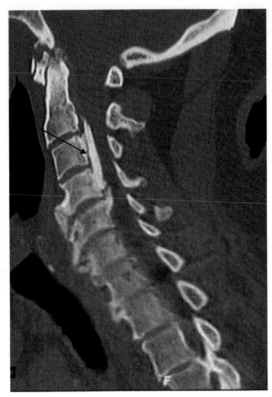

Fig. 8. CT scan depicting OPLL in the cervical spine causing narrowing of the central canal. (*Courtesy of* Pietrowski D, MSN ACNP ONP-C, Chicago, IL.)

or deformity. Palpate the spine itself and the paraspinal musculature for pain. Upper and lower extremities are checked from a motor and sensory perspective. Distinct signs are assessed, including

- Lhermitte sign (forward flexion of neck producing a lightning feeling in the extremities)
- Hoffman's Sign (abnormal flexion of the digits after manually flicking on fingernail)
- Sustained clonus (rapid flexion of the foot resulting in involuntary beats of the foot)
- Hyperreflexia (of the upper and/or lower extremities)
- Babinski (stimulation of the sole of the foot resulting in a fanning of the toes)

Diagnostic imaging is helpful in locating the area and cause of compression and the effects on the neural structures. Plain radiographs assess for bony alignment and spondyloarthropathies. CT scan can further elicit abnormalities, size of the canal, and the presence of OPLL. The degree of spinal cord compression and injury is best assessed on the T2-weighted images of an MRI. White signal within a dark cord is indicative of spinal cord damage or myelomalacia. If the amount of compression has progressed to causing myelomalacia, this indicates more permanent injury and decreases the chance of deficit recovery.[28] Patients with myelopathy must understand that surgical treatment is to arrest further decline and may not necessarily improve the symptoms.

Lumbar stenosis

Narrowing of the canal in the lumbar region is more concerning for nerve compression versus spinal cord compression due to the termination of the cord at the L1 level. A variable combination of disc degeneration, arthritic changes in the superior and inferior vertebral bodies, and facet arthropathy can decrease the diameter of the lumbar canal.[29] Other concerns are for disc herniations, facet cysts, and lipomatosis as contributing factors. Initial symptoms present as back discomfort or stiffness usually associated with activity or ambulation. When nerves are irritated or compressed, patients can feel radicular changes in the legs, including pain, alterations in sensation, and weakness. Neurogenic claudication is the amount of stenosis and compression, which limits a patient's ability to walk distances.[30] A forward stooped posture while ambulating can relieve nerve compression (positive shopping cart sign).

Most patients present when symptoms disrupt activities of daily living and they notice a decrease in quality of life. A forward stooped posture (sagittal imbalance) and tenderness to palpation are common. Range of motion is decreased in all planes. A description of extremity symptoms, including pain or sensation changes, follows a radicular pattern based on the level and laterality of compression. Foot drop due to weakness should be ruled out. Straight leg raise testing can further confirm irritation of a nerve root and can be performed supine or seated.[31]

Plain radiographs check for degenerative disc disease, fractures, spondylolisthesis, and any dynamic instability with flexion and extension views. For a better understanding of the neuroelements, disc pathology, and cysts, MRIs are ordered (**Fig. 9**). On occasion there may be a neurologic differential diagnosis that is concerning for the lower extremities, and EMG/NCS can be ordered to differentiate a nerve root compression from a peripheral nerve problem. This can be the case in foot drop when ruling out L5 compression versus a compression of the peroneal nerve. Vascular disease also can mimic claudication symptoms and can be picked up with a simple distal pulse check. Patients with this presentation should be worked-up further by a vascular team.

Fractures

Compression fractures due to osteoporosis are a concern in the orthopedic and primary care community due to the current epidemic that is facing the American

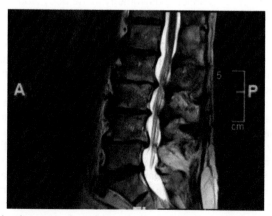

Fig. 9. MRI of the lumbar spine depicting stenosis at multiple levels due to degenerative disc disease. (*Courtesy of* Pietrowski D, MSN ACNP ONP-C, Chicago, IL.)

population; 44 million are affected by osteoporosis in the United States, causing expenditures to exceed $19 billion annually.[32] Risk factors include white women, age over 50, and post-menopause. Modifiable risks, such as smoking and obesity, affect the ability to absorb calcium. Other concerns are for certain medications, such as steroids, antidepressants, and diabetes drugs, that also alter bone health.

Osteoporotic compression fractures occur mostly through the body of a vertebrae. They typically are a source of axial back pain without neurologic deficits. Occasionally a patient presents with nerve irritation and radiating pain. Serial radiographs are taken to check for signs of healing, alignment, and any new deformity that may occur, because one of the major risks to a new vertebral compression fracture is a previous fracture in the same region.[33] MRI can confirm acuity of the fracture, because bony edema lights up on short-tau inversion recovery (STIR) sequencing.

Traumatic fractures are related to the mechanism of injury. If an injury entails high-energy axial loading of the spine with flexion, a burst fracture is likely. A burst fracture involves disruption of the posterior elements of the vertebra and is deemed unstable because loose bony fragments can retropulse and compress neuroelements. A chance fracture is seen in motor vehicle accidents due to high speed and seat belts. This fracture involves flexion and distraction, fracturing the vertebral body, and disrupting the posterior ligaments. A baseline motor and neurologic examination is important in understanding any progression of deficit and deciding on a treatment plan.

Scoliosis

The 3-dimensional rotation of the spine defines the term scoliosis. It is an understanding of the underlying cause that determines treatment options. Idiopathic scoliosis presents during adolescence, with an incidence of 0.47% to 5.2% in the literature.[34] Congenital scoliosis is caused by a malformation or defect of the vertebrae in the spine that causes deformity. Neuromuscular scoliosis can be more rapidly progressing because the curvature itself can be caused by conditions, such as cerebral palsy or muscular dystrophy. Degenerative scoliosis occurs later in life due to the asymmetric degeneration of the spinal components. Due to the multicomponent aspect of the deformity, degenerative scoliosis is a significant cause of pain and disability.[35]

Patient presentation at a clinic for idiopathic scoliosis may be due to an examination by a school nurse or parents noticing asymmetry in the body (such as a height difference in the shoulders). Teenagers typically do not present in pain. There may be noted truncal shift, leg length differences, and rib rotation on Adams forward bending test. To perform this test, a patient begins standing straight with arms stretched forward. A patient bends forward, and a scoliometer is used to measure the rotation of the spine. Serial radiographs are used to monitor the progression of the curvature by using Cobb angles. Radiographs also are used to understand bone maturity with the use of Risser staging and open triradiate cartilage. A hand radiograph is also helpful in understanding skeletal maturity. Understanding the peak growth velocity takes into account the beginning of menarche.

Due to maturity of the spine, degenerative scoliosis can present with significant pain and radicular symptoms as a result of the amount of compression on the central or neuroforaminal canals. The patient notices changes in ambulation and stamina with activities and eventually a decrease in quality of life.[36] The symptoms usually occur in a radicular pattern or can present as a form of claudication. Decreased range of motion with pain is a hallmark sign. A forward stooped posture, or sagittal imbalance, not only is due to the deformity but also is the result of a patient trying to unload the posterior elements of the spine, taking pressure off the nerves. Plain radiographs assist in understanding the cause of the deformity, and an MRI helps decipher which neuroelements are involved in the symptomatic presentation.

MANAGEMENT OF SPINAL PATHOLOGIES

Treatment of spine patients through the continuum has made great strides from both nonoperative and operative perspectives. With the current opioid crisis plaguing the United States, patients no longer are treated with narcotics as a first line of pharmaceutical management for spine pain. A position statement by the National Association of Orthopaedic Nurses cites the need for increased provider and patient education along with the need for multimodal and alternative therapies.[37] Combining medications, such as nonsteroidal anti-inflammatory drugs (NSAIDs) and muscle relaxants, has proved better tolerated and more effective.[38] Other pharmacologic therapies include the use of acetaminophen, cyclooxygenase-2 inhibitors, and neurotransmitter inhibitors.[39] From an anesthetic perspective, a trial of blocks (ie, epidural and never root) and intraoperative surgical site injections can make a difference in early mobilization and recovery.

Osteoporosis management in the early stages focuses on maintaining strong healthy bone, while preventing fragility fractures. Women over age 65 are recommended to get a bone density screen (DEXA) and those who have an increased risk should have one completed sooner.[40] Assessment tools, such as fracture risk assessment tool (FRAX) scores, can guide the treating team in deciding when to order a dual-energy x-ray absorptiometry scan and further laboratory testing. Studies have concluded that the use of bisphosphonate therapy specifically in the spine is associated with fewer fractures compared with placebo.[41] An open discussion among patient, orthopedic team, primary care, and endocrinology can prevent fragility fractures while helping a patient modify risks, such as smoking, immobility, alcoholism, and low vitamin D.[42]

There is a specific role that physical therapy plays in the treatment of spine pathologies. Early intervention from a physical therapist has shown to improve pain intensity, quality of life, and overall disability.[43] Prescriptions need to specify diagnosis and give direction as to the type of therapies that would maximize the benefit versus a generic evaluate and treat. Muscular stabilization, stretching, and protraction are helpful in the pathologies of the cervical spine, whereas core strengthening and postural strengthening are cornerstones for the lumbar spine.[44–46] It is imperative that a home exercise program be incorporated into daily exercise as a form of long-term management.

Long-term hospitalizations and skilled nursing facility stays have been found to increase complication rates, decrease quality of life, and increase financial burden. Patients are leaving the hospital on same day after surgical procedures, such as discectomies and anterior cervical discectomy and fusions (ACDF), with similarly low admission rates compared with those of admitted patients.[47] Ambulation after a spine procedure happens the day of surgery versus waiting to ambulate on the next day. Early ambulation has shown to improve pain and disability.[48] The simple act of walking has improved rates of healing while recovering quality of life, mood, and satisfaction.[49]

INNOVATIONS IN SPINE CARE

Trends in treatment of spine conditions have focused on safety, cost containment, and satisfaction. These 3 outcomes focus not only on the patient but also on the health care team. Recurring themes in surgical procedures focus on smaller incisions, decreased length of stay, and the use of technology to attain those goals. Studies regarding spine care have worked to quantify these goals in the form of successful patient outcomes.

The use of robotics in spine surgery has focused on precision surgical techniques with the goal of perfecting instrumentation placement and decreasing operative complications. Robotics also plays a role in minimally invasive surgery (MIS). Smaller incisions, decreased dissection, and decreased instability of the spine have made MIS easily marketable. The increased development and use of ambulatory surgical centers (ASCs) for spine promotes discharge on the same calendar day. These 3 themes are some of the driving forces that are reshaping the surgical options for the future.

Robotics

As with the use of computer-assisted surgeries in the 1990s, the evolution of technology has progressed to the application of robotics in the operating room. When placing instrumentation at various angles in the spine, such as screws in pedicles, there is a margin of human error, with concerns of injury to the neuroelements and vasculature. The goal of robotics is to improve the accuracy of instrumentation placement and decrease radiation to the patient and the surgical team, resulting in improved outcomes, such as length of stay, patient satisfaction, and complication rates.[50]

The current robotic technology strives to decrease surgeon error by providing live feedback in guiding the placement of instrumentation. A CT scan is required either preoperatively or intraoperatively and registered to guide the robot. The robot cannot account for any bone that needs to be removed during a decompressive procedure and thus a revised scan may be needed at the time of surgery. The unit itself is fastened to the patient with bone attachments that allow it to cannulate pedicles.

Future software is being developed to facilitate spinal correction (deformity), with the use of patient-specific contoured rods.[51] Robots also are being developed that not only drill but also remove bone to help in decompressive type procedures. The potential use of MRI can assist the surgical team in providing a map of the neuroelements during the surgical case and decreasing radiation exposure if further intraoperative CTs are required once bony elements are removed.[52] But it is the 3-dimensional analytics of these robots that assist with planning, notably in minimally invasive cases, adding another tool to the surgeons toolbox.

Minimally Invasive Spine Surgery

The theory behind MIS for spine surgery is that a smaller incision has the benefits of decreased blood loss, length of hospital stay, and pain.[53] The public marketing of this surgical option has patients asking about a swift return to activities while decreasing the cost burden (both direct and indirect). Studies have compared MIS techniques with traditional open incisions and have found decreased length of stay, postoperative pain, and use of narcotic medications.[54] Furthermore, MIS procedures, such as decompressions and transforaminal lumbar interbody fusions, have been shown to increase satisfaction rates through disability scores.[55,56]

As more clinical settings offer MIS as an option, patients need to be educated about criteria and the surgical implications. With the smaller MIS incision, the surgeon may employ the use of navigation or robotics to decrease the disruption of a patient's anatomy while achieving goals of decompression and/or stabilization. Smaller puncture-type incisions can be made at multiple sites for longer constructs while also using percutaneous instrumentation, decreasing the amount of trauma to surrounding tissues.[57]

Postoperative variations for the MIS patient include reduced rehabilitation and the decrease use of custom orthotic bracing. Prehabilitation and maintenance of stabilization exercises postoperatively have replaced months of postoperative rehabilitation and custom bracing. As the length of stay has decreased for this patient population, an opportunity for same-day discharges has grown in cases, such as discectomies for disc herniations and anterior cervical discectomy and fusions. The trend of outpatient spine surgery has increased as has the use of ASCs.

Ambulatory Surgical Centers

ASCs have become part of many strategic plans due to efficiency in the operating rooms, quicker turnover of cases, and greater access for surgeons and patients.[58] With the push for same day discharges due to decreased reimbursement, these centers have become a hub for spine surgeries allowing for a reduction of costs to multiple providers as they allow for surgeons to work with the same team. The concern lies in making sure that the patient population is optimized as these standalone facilities do not plan for long term observation, such as outpatient surgery. Caution is given to patients with multiple comorbidities and cases that require increased time in the operating room as the risks for complications can be critical.

By definition, a patient who is admitted as an outpatient needs to be discharged within 23 hours. ASCs discharge patients from their facilities on the same day. Some surgeons still find comfort in outpatient surgery in the hospital setting as it allows for postoperative assessment. The major concerns are for bleeding at the surgical site along with neurologic compromise. Smaller surgeries, such as single-level decompressions, have increased in the true outpatient setting to 68.5% as well as discectomies (46.7%).[59] From an ASC perspective, the increases are modest in the same time frame when looking at single-level decompressions (10.6%). Patient selection and the use of protocols will optimize safety in ASCs leading to increased numbers in the future.[60]

SUMMARY

The push for patient outcomes and financial implications on spine care has changed both short-term and long-term treatment plans for similar diagnoses that have been managed for years. Patients are continuing to educate themselves on newer technologies while providers are balancing evidence-based practice with new techniques and technology. Many innovations that are arising in spine care need to be assessed and evaluated from quality and patient safety perspectives. Although the natural history of spinal disorders will continue with the aging process, measures to increase quality of life while limiting disability will continue to be the cornerstone of innovation.

DISCLOSURE

The author has nothing to disclose.

REFERENCES

1. Waterman BR, Belmont PJ Jr, Schoenfeld AJ. Low back pain in the United States: incidence and risk factors for presentation in the emergency setting. Spine J 2012;12(1):63–70.
2. Shmagel A, Foley R, Ibrahim H. Epidemiology of chronic low back pain in US adults: data from the 2009-2010 national health and nutrition examination survey. Arthritis Care Res 2016;68(11):1688–94.
3. Wei Q, Zhang X, Zhou C, et al. Roles of large aggregating proteoglycans in human intervertebral disc degeneration. Connect Tissue Res 2019;60(3):209–18.

4. Petersen T, Laslett M, Juhl C. Clinical classification in low back pain: best-evidence diagnostic rules based on systematic reviews. BMC Musculoskelet Disord 2017;18(1):188.

5. Reidler JS, Jain A, Khanna AJ. Cervical spine trauma. The Spine Handbook. New York: Oxford University Press; 2018. p. 147.

6. Joaquim AF, Ghizoni E, Tedeschi H, et al. Radiological evaluation of cervical spine involvement in rheumatoid arthritis. Neurosurg Focus 2015;38(4):E4.

7. Patel DR, Kinsella E. Evaluation and management of lower back pain in young athletes. Transl Pediatr 2017;6(3):225.

8. Halati FN, Vajhi A, Molazem M, et al. Are magnetic resonance imaging or radiographic findings correlated with clinical prognosis in spinal cord neuropathy? Paper presented at: Veterinary Research Forum. Urmia Iran, Summer 2016.

9. Jain M, Sahu NK, Naik S, et al. Symptomatic Tarlov cyst in cervical spine. BMJ Case Rep 2018;11(1) [pii:e228051].

10. Splendiani A, D'Orazio F, Patriarca L, et al. Imaging of post-operative spine in intervertebral disc pathology. Musculoskelet Surg 2017;101(1):75–84.

11. Tobert DG, Harris MB. Degenerative lumbar spinal stenosis and spondylolisthesis. In: Katz JN, Blauwet CA, Schoenfeld AJ, editors. Principles of orthopedic practice for primary care providers. New York: Springer; 2018. p. 47–59.

12. Alsaleh K, Ho D, Rosas-Arellano MP, et al. Radiographic assessment of degenerative lumbar spinal stenosis: is MRI superior to CT? Eur Spine J 2017;26(2):362–7.

13. Divi SN, Saitta B, Clair JS, et al. Diagnostic modalities and nonoperative treatment of lumbar spinal stenosis. Seminars in Spine Surgery 2019;31(3):100710.

14. Maher C, Underwood M, Buchbinder R. Non-specific low back pain. Lancet 2017;389(10070):736–47.

15. Williams JS, Ng N, Peltzer K, et al. Risk factors and disability associated with low back pain in older adults in low-and middle-income countries. Results from the WHO study on global AGEing and adult health (SAGE). PLoS One 2015;10(6):e0127880.

16. Hur JW, Park D-H, Lee J-B, et al. Guidelines for cauda equina syndrome management. Journal of Neurointensive Care 2019;2(1):14–6.

17. Yang S-D, Chen Q, Ding W-Y. Cauda equina syndrome due to vigorous back massage with spinal manipulation in a patient with pre-existing lumbar disc herniation: a case report and literature review. Am J Phys Med Rehabil 2018;97(4):e23–6.

18. Yates JR, Jones CS, Stokes OM, et al. Incomplete cauda equina syndrome secondary to haemorrhage within a Tarlov cyst. BMJ Case Rep 2017;2017 [pii: bcr-2017-219890].

19. Rider IS, Marra EM. Cauda equina and conus medullaris syndromes. In: StatPearls [Internet]. Treasure Island (FL): StatPearls Publishing; 2019.

20. McDonald BT, Lucas JA. Spondylolysis. In: StatPearls [Internet]. Treasure Island (FL): StatPearls Publishing; 2018.

21. Berger RG, Doyle SM. Spondylolysis 2019 update. Curr Opin Pediatr 2019;31(1):61–8.

22. Nielsen E, Andras LM, Skaggs DL. Diagnosis of spondylolysis and spondylolisthesis is delayed six months after seeing nonorthopedic providers. Spine Deform 2018;6(3):263–6.

23. Riley PM, Micheli LJ. Back pain in the young athlete. In: Caine D, Purcell L, editors. Injury in pediatric and adolescent sports. New York: Springer; 2016. p. 135–47.

24. Matsunaga S, Sakou T, Morizono Y, et al. Natural history of degenerative spondy-lolisthesis. Pathogenesis and natural course of the slippage. Spine 1990;15(11): 1204–10.

25. Graham RB, Hashmi S, Maslak JP, et al. Lumbar deformity spondylolisthesis (moderate–high grade) complication. In: Mummaneni PV, Park P, Crawford CH III, et al, editors. Spinal deformity. New York: Springer; 2018. p. 291–300.

26. Davies BM, Mowforth OD, Smith EK, et al. Degenerative cervical myelopathy. BMJ 2018;360:k186.

27. Hou X, Sun C, Liu X, et al. Clinical features of thoracic spinal stenosis-associated myelopathy: a retrospective analysis of 427 cases. Clin Spine Surg 2016; 29(2):86–9.

28. Nouri A, Tetreault L, Nori S, et al. Congenital cervical spine stenosis in a global cohort of patients with degenerative cervical myelopathy: a report based on a MRI diagnostic criterion. Spine J 2017;17(10):S134.

29. Lee SY, Kim T-H, Oh JK, et al. Lumbar stenosis: a recent update by review of liter-ature. Asian Spine J 2015;9(5):818.

30. Markman JD, Gewandter JS, Frazer ME, et al. Evaluation of outcome measures for neurogenic claudication: a patient-centered approach. Neurology 2015; 85(14):1250–6.

31. Colangelo T, Koerner JD, Vaccaro AR. Chapter 2. Lower back pain in adults. In: Koerner JD, Vaccaro AR, Kim DH, editors. Differential Diagnosis in Spine Surgery. New Delhi, India: Jaypee Brothers Medical Publishers; 2016. p. 19–32.

32. Osteoporosis epidemic. Available at: https://www.ownthebone.org/OTB/About/ Why_Own_the_Bone.aspx. Accessed May 15, 2019.

33. Lee SJ, Graffy PM, Zea RD, et al. Future osteoporotic fracture risk related to lum-bar vertebral trabecular attenuation measured at routine body CT. J Bone Miner Res 2018;33(5):860–7.

34. Konieczny MR, Senyurt H, Krauspe R. Epidemiology of adolescent idiopathic scoliosis. J Child Orthop 2013;7(1):3–9.

35. Shaffrey CI, Smith JS, Ames CP, et al. Introduction. Adult spinal deformity. Neuro-surg Focus 2017;43(6):E1.

36. Pellisé F, Vila-Casademunt A, Ferrer M, et al. Impact on health related quality of life of adult spinal deformity (ASD) compared with other chronic conditions. Eur Spine J 2015;24(1):3–11.

37. Combs B, Hughes MM, Ariagno J, et al. Opioid epidemic. Orthop Nurs 2019; 38(2):92–4.

38. Patel HD, Uppin R, Naidu AR, et al. Efficacy and safety of combination of NSAIDs and muscle relaxants in the management of acute low back pain. Pain Ther 2019; 8(1):121–32.

39. Anderson I, Alger J. The tightrope walk: pain management and opioid steward-ship. Orthop Nurs 2019;38(2):111–5.

40. Viswanathan M, Reddy S, Berkman N, et al. Screening to prevent osteoporotic fractures: updated evidence report and systematic review for the US preventive services task ForceUSPSTF evidence report: screening to prevent osteoporotic FracturesUSPSTF evidence report: screening to prevent osteoporotic fractures. JAMA 2018;319(24):2532–51.

41. Adler RA, El-Hajj Fuleihan G, Bauer DC, et al. Managing osteoporosis in patients on long-term bisphosphonate treatment: report of a task force of the American Society for Bone and Mineral Research. J Bone Miner Res 2016;31(1):16–35.

42. Pisani P, Renna MD, Conversano F, et al. Major osteoporotic fragility fractures: risk factor updates and societal impact. World J Orthop 2016;7(3):171.

43. Fritz JM, Magel JS, McFadden M, et al. Early physical therapy vs usual care in patients with recent-onset low back pain: a randomized clinical trial. JAMA 2015;314(14):1459–67.

44. Abdelraouf OR, Abdel-aziem AA. The relationship between core endurance and back dysfunction in collegiate male athletes with and without nonspecific low back pain. Int J Sports Phys Ther 2016;11(3):337.

45. Kumar T, Kumar S, Nezamuddin M, et al. Efficacy of core muscle strengthening exercise in chronic low back pain patients. J Back Musculoskelet Rehabil 2015; 28(4):699–707.

46. Chang W-D, Lin H-Y, Lai P-T. Core strength training for patients with chronic low back pain. J Phys Ther Sci 2015;27(3):619–22.

47. Shenoy K, Adenikinju A, Dweck E, et al. Friday, September 28, 2018 10: 30 AM–12: 00 PM abstracts: complications of cervical spine surgery: 155. Same day discharge after anterior cervical discectomy and fusion in suitable patients has similarly low readmission rates as admitted patients. Spine J 2018;18(8):S77.

48. Adogwa O, Elsamadicy AA, Fialkoff J, et al. Assessing the effectiveness of routine use of post-operative in-patient physical therapy services. J Spine Surg 2017; 3(2):149.

49. Kalisch BJ, Lee S, Dabney BW. Outcomes of inpatient mobilization: a literature review. J Clin Nurs 2014;23(11–12):1486–501.

50. Divi S, Pollster S, Ramos E, et al. The current role of robotic technology in spine surgery. Oper Tech Orthop 2017;27(4):275–82.

51. Malham GM, Wells-Quinn T. What should my hospital buy next?—guidelines for the acquisition and application of imaging, navigation, and robotics for spine surgery. J Spine Surg 2019;5(1):155.

52. Overley SC, Cho SK, Mehta AI, et al. Navigation and robotics in spinal surgery: where are we now? Neurosurgery 2017;80(3S):S86–99.

53. Lee MJ, Mok J, Patel P. Transforaminal lumbar interbody fusion: traditional open versus minimally invasive techniques. J Am Acad Orthop Surg 2018;26(4): 124–31.

54. Skovrlj B, Belton P, Zarzour H, et al. Perioperative outcomes in minimally invasive lumbar spine surgery: a systematic review. World J Orthop 2015;6(11):996.

55. Nerland US, Jakola AS, Solheim O, et al. Minimally invasive decompression versus open laminectomy for central stenosis of the lumbar spine: pragmatic comparative effectiveness study. BMJ 2015;350:h1603.

56. Kim J-S, Jung B, Lee S-H. Instrumented minimally invasive spinal-transforaminal lumbar interbody fusion (MIS-TLIF). Clin Spine Surg 2018;31(6):E302–9.

57. Keric N, Eum DJ, Afghanyar F, et al. Evaluation of surgical strategy of conventional vs. percutaneous robot-assisted spinal trans-pedicular instrumentation in spondylodiscitis. J Robot Surg 2017;11(1):17–25.

58. Nandyala SV, Bono CM. The ultimate decrease in length of stay: Outpatient spine surgery. Seminars in Spine Surgery 2019;30(1):20–4.

59. Idowu O, Boyadjian H, Shi L, et al. Trend of spine surgeries in the outpatient hospital setting versus ambulatory surgical center. Spine J 2017;17(10):S204.

60. Patel DV, Yoo JS, Karmarkar SS, et al. Minimally invasive lumbar decompression in an ambulatory surgery center. J Spine Surg 2019;5(Suppl 2):S166–73.

Fighting the Epidemic
Bone Health and Osteoporosis

Debra L. Sietsema, MSN, PhD[a,b,*]

KEYWORDS

- Osteoporosis • Bone health • Osteoporosis management • Osteoporosis prevention
- Osteoporosis treatment • Fracture risk • Bone mineral density

KEY POINTS

- Osteoporosis is a growing epidemic, resulting in a public health problem, affecting the quality of life of millions of people.
- Fragility fractures frequently occur after age 50 and are a personal, health care, and socioeconomic burden.
- Osteoporosis can be prevented, screened, diagnosed, and treated before fractures occur.
- Bone health care, including assessment, diagnosis, treatment, and counseling, should be done as part of standard nursing care.
- Identification and treatment must follow fragility fractures to prevent subsequent fractures.

OSTEOPOROSIS AND BONE HEALTH INTRODUCTION

Bone health is defined as a public health issue with an emphasis on prevention and early intervention to promote strong bones and prevent fractures and their consequences.[1] Osteoporosis is a common disease that is characterized by low bone mass, deterioration of bone tissue, and disruption of bone microarchitecture resulting in an increased risk of fracture.[2] With an aging population and longer life span, osteoporosis is increasingly becoming an epidemic, making this a major public health problem that can be fought by nurses.

PREVALENCE

At the time of the last US census in 2010, the overall prevalence of osteoporosis in adults aged 50 and older was approximately 10.2 million. The prevalence was significantly higher in women (16.5%) than men (5.1%).[3,4] The overall prevalence of low bone mass was approximately 45 million adults. The prevalence of low bone mass was higher in women (52.6%) than in men (35.6%).[3,4] This osteoporosis and low

[a] Bone Health Clinical Operations, The CORE Institute®, Phoenix, AZ, USA; [b] Grants and Education, MORE Foundation, Phoenix, AZ, USA
* 33575 North Dove Lakes Drive, Unit 1017, Cave Creek, AZ 85331.
E-mail address: debra.sietsema@gmail.com

Nurs Clin N Am 55 (2020) 193–202
https://doi.org/10.1016/j.cnur.2020.02.002
0029-6465/20/© 2020 Elsevier Inc. All rights reserved.

bone mass population is expected to increase to 121.3 million by 2025.[5,6] Despite the increasing prevalence of osteoporosis, national Healthcare Effectiveness Data and Information Set measures demonstrate that less than one-third of people after fracture have received testing or treatment.[7] This creates a substantial treatment gap that nurses must fight against.

ECONOMIC BURDEN

Osteoporosis and fragility fractures are associated with increased health care utilization, including hospitalization stays, physician office visits, and pharmacy use.[3,8] Health care costs continue to rise related to osteoporosis. Total aggregate direct costs (ambulatory care, inpatient, prescription, other health care costs) for all persons were $73.6 billion from 2012 to 2014, a rise of 118% from the $28.1 billion in 1998 to 2000, in 2014 dollars.[9] The greatest change in average per-person cost was for prescriptions, rising from $1771 in 1998 to 2000 to $3,494, in 2014 dollars, an increase of 97%.[9]

OSTEOPOROSIS CONSEQUENCES

Osteoporosis develops gradually, without warning signs or symptoms. Because the first warning sign is frequently a fracture, osteoporosis is often called a "silent disease" or "silent thief." It literally steals bone mass without giving any indication until a fragility fracture occurs. Fragility fractures are defined as those occurring spontaneously, following a fall from a standing height or less, or with minimal trauma. Fractures do not normally occur in these situations in people with healthy bones. Most fragility fractures occur in those who are not osteoporotic determined by bone mineral density (BMD) t-score. An osteoporosis fracture is defined as those occurring after the diagnosis of osteoporosis based on a t-score of ≤ -2.5. The most common sites of fragility fracture are the vertebral compression fracture, hip, and distal radius. These can have devastating personal and societal consequences, including pain, decreased quality of life, increased disability-adjusted life span, loss of independence, financial burden, and even death.[10,11]

BONE FRAGILITY PATHOGENESIS

Bone strength is determined by its density and quality.[12] Bone is a living organ and has continuous modeling (construction) and remodeling (reconstruction). Bone modeling occurs when bone is deposited without previous bone resorption. During bone remodeling, resorption by osteoclasts precedes bone formation by osteoblasts.[12] The bone mass is modeled and remodeled during growth from birth to early adulthood, reaching peak bone mass by approximately age 30. Peak bone mass is determined mostly by genetic factors, health during growth, nutrition, endocrine status, gender, and physical activity. Subsequently, bone loss starts. Bone resorption is essential for the excavation of a marrow cavity and the development of cortical and trabecular bone during growth.[12] In adults, osteocytes sense bone deformation, microcracks, and the resorption that removes damaged bone, signaling the need for adaptive remodeling and formation restoration of new bone.[12] BMD decreases when the resorption is more than the formation rate. The death of osteocytes in estrogen deficiency, during corticosteroid therapy, in advancing age, or after damage to bone is associated with a loss of bone strength before any bone loss.[12] An imbalance between resorption and formation with increased resorption during menopause and aging causes an increased risk for fracture. Other secondary risk factors may also affect remodeling, reduce bone quality, or disrupt microarchitectural integrity.

ASSESSMENT/SCREENING

BMD assessment, along with a detailed history and physical examination, vertebral fracture assessment, when appropriate, and fracture risk assessment tool (FRAX), are completed to establish an individual patient's fracture risk.

The goal of osteoporosis screening is prevention and to identify persons at increased risk of fragility fracture and initiate intervention to minimize risks. The gold standard for screening is obtaining a BMD using dual-energy x-ray absorptiometry (DXA). BMD is grams per square centimeter of calcification in the scanned bone. See **Table 1** for the indications for BMD testing.[13] Vertebral compression fractures are common in older adults and often are undiagnosed. A vertebral fracture assessment, available on most DXA machines, or lateral spine radiograph may be done with the baseline BMD screening or for the following indications[13]:

- Women aged ≥70 years or men aged ≥80 years
- Historical height loss: difference between the current height and peak height at age 20 ≥4 cm
- Prospective height loss: difference between the current height and a previously documented height measurement of ≥2 cm
- Self-reported but undocumented prior vertebral fracture
- Recent or ongoing long-term glucocorticoid treatment (equivalent to ≥5 mg of prednisone or equivalent per day for ≥3 months)

In addition to BMD, clinical risk factors should be determined. A FRAX can be obtained at www.shef.ac.uk/FRAX. The weight of clinical risk factors with or without BMD are incorporated in the FRAX algorithms. It measures the 10-year risk of major osteoporotic and hip fractures. Fracture risk probabilities have been determined for several countries. Clinical risk factors used to determine FRAX 10-year fracture probability include the following:

- Current age
- Sex
- A prior osteoporotic fracture (including clinical and asymptomatic vertebral fractures)

Table 1 Indications for bone mineral density (BMD) testing	
Gender/Age	**Condition**
Women ≥65 y	Healthy
Men ≥70 y	Healthy
Post or perimenopausal women <65 y and men <70 y	Risk factors such as • Low body weight • Prior fragility fracture • High-risk medication use • Disease or condition associated with bone loss
Adults	• With a fragility fracture • Disease or condition associated with low bone mass or bone loss • Taking medications associated with low bone mass or bone loss • Being considered for osteoporosis pharmacologic therapy • To monitor treatment effect of osteoporosis treatment • Evidence of bone loss would lead to treatment

- Body mass index
- Oral glucocorticoids $\geq$5 mg/d of prednisone for >3 months (ever)
- Rheumatoid arthritis
- Parental history of hip fracture
- Secondary causes of osteoporosis
- Being a past or current smoker
- Alcohol intake ($\geq$3 drinks/d)
- Femoral neck BMD (optional)

Additional risk factors should be assessed. Behavioral lifestyle factors, including nutrition and supplement intake, physical activity, smoking, and alcohol use, should be determined. A thorough medical and medication history should be taken to determine possible causes of secondary osteoporosis. Comorbidity causes of secondary osteoporosis in adults is well documented according to genetic endocrine, gastrointestinal hematological, musculoskeletal, neurologic, rheumatologic, autoimmune, and other diseases/conditions.[14,15] Drugs that can affect bone health include, but are not limited to, antiseizure, aromatase inhibitors, chemotherapy/immunosuppressants, Depo-Provera, glucocorticoids, gonadotropin-releasing hormone agents, heparin, lithium, proton pump inhibitors, selective serotonin reuptake inhibitors, thiazolidinediones, and thyroid hormone.[14] Prior fragility fractures after age 50 should be recorded.

Falls are the cause of most fragility fractures. The frequency of falls during the previous year should be assessed. Environmental, medical, and pharmaceutical risk factors increasing the propensity for falls should be determined.

CLINICAL FINDINGS

Fragility fractures and their complications may be the first clinical consequence of osteoporosis. A recent fracture in a person older than 50 years with or without trauma suggests that further assessment is needed. Fractures may cause chronic pain, disability, and death.[11,16]

Loss of height can be the result of vertebral compression fracture(s). Using a stadiometer, height should be followed serially by a health care professional. If not measured routinely, a comparison can be made to the person's recollection of her or his height when they obtained their first drivers' license as a young adult or his or her tallest height.[17,18] Height loss of 2 cm or more when measured serially or 4 cm or more when compared with young adult height could be a sign that vertebral compression fracture(s) may be present.[15] With multiple vertebral compression fractures, dorsal kyphosis can be objectively detected by increased occiput-to-wall distance. Positional restrictions may ensue. Vertebral thoracic fractures may result in restrictive lung disease and secondary heart problems. Vertebral lumbar fractures may alter abdominal anatomy, affecting the gastrointestinal system causing a variety of related complaints. Additional assessment can include psychosocial issues of prolonged disability, poor self-image, social isolation, and depression.

LABORATORY STUDIES

Laboratory studies to rule out secondary osteoporosis and to assist in pharmacotherapy selection are listed in **Box 1**.[14-16,19] In addition, bone turnover markers (BTMs) indicate the rate of bone formation and resorption, which may provide information on fracture risk, and can be used to demonstrate the response to treatments. Following antiresorptive therapy, the greater the decrease in BTM, the larger the

---

Box 1
Laboratory tests

First-line Secondary Osteoporosis Screening
   Complete blood cell count
   Chemistry, serum, including calcium, phosphorus, magnesium, total protein, albumin, liver
   enzymes (alanine aminotransferase and aspartate amino transferase), alkaline phosphatase,
   creatinine, and electrolytes
   25-hydroxyvitamin D, serum

Second-line Secondary Osteoporosis Screening
   C-telopeptide, serum
   Aminoterminal propeptide of type I procollagen, serum
   Parathyroid hormone
   Thyroid-stimulating hormone and free T4
   Total testosterone (men)
   24-h urine collection for calcium sodium, and creatinine excretion

Secondary Osteoporosis Screening if There is Clinical Suspicion
   Acid-base studies
   Erythrocyte sedimentation rate
   Homocysteine
   Iron and ferritin levels
   Prolactin
   Thyrotropin, serum
   Tissue transglutaminase antibodies (immunoglobulin [Ig]A and IgG) for suspected celiac
   disease
   Tryptase, serum, urine N-methylhistamine, or other tests for mastocytosis
   Serum protein electrophoresis for suspected myeloma
   Urinary protein electrophoresis
   Urinary free cortisol or other tests for suspected adrenal hypersecretion
   Urinary histamine

---

reduction in fracture risk.[13] Serum aminoterminal propeptide of type I procollagen and C-telopeptide should be used to measure bone formation and resorption, respectively.[19]

DIAGNOSIS

The World Health Organization (WHO) has defined and provides the diagnostic categories for osteoporosis based on DXA measurements[13,14,19] (**Table 2**). In addition to the WHO diagnostic category using t-score ≤-2.5, osteoporosis can be clinically diagnosed in individuals who have had a fragility fracture, irrespective of BMD.[20] Osteoporosis can be diagnosed for those who have experienced a fragility hip fracture and for those who have low bone mass by BMD who sustain a fragility vertebral, proximal humerus, pelvis, or in some cases, distal forearm fracture.[20] Also, osteoporosis should be diagnosed for those who have an elevated fracture risk based on FRAX.[20]

PRIMARY AND SECONDARY PREVENTION AND TREATMENT OPTIONS

Several recommended interventions and treatments, including lifestyle behaviors of adequate nutrition; intake of calcium and vitamin D; regular weight-bearing, core and muscle-strengthening exercise; cessation of tobacco use and excessive alcohol intake; and decreasing risk of falling are fundamental for osteoporosis prevention or treatment.[21] Counseling regarding risk of osteoporosis and related fractures is essential. In addition, pharmacologic treatment may be recommended. Although there are

Table 2 Osteoporosis categories based on DXA BMD	
Category	**Bone Mass *t*-Score**
Normal	≥ -1.0 SD
Low bone mass (osteopenia)	< -1.0 and > -2.5 SD
Osteoporosis	≤ -2.5
Severe osteoporosis	< -2.5 and ≥ 1 fragility fracture

Abbreviations: BMD, bone mineral density; DXA, dual-energy x-ray absorptiometry.

several guidelines available, this author finds the American Orthopedic Association Own the Bone,[22] American Association of Clinical Endocrinologists Medical Guidelines,[14] and Clinician's Guide to Prevention and Treatment of Osteoporosis[15] to be congruent with orthopedic nursing practice.

One way to promote bone health and decrease the risk of osteoporosis is to maximize peak bone mass. Forty percent of adult skeletal calcium is accumulated in the 4 years during peak height growth during adolescence, making adolescence a critical time for bone development.[23] Lifestyle behaviors can moderately increase peak bone mass. Lifestyle factors can account for 20% to 40% of the variance in peak bone mass, whereas gender, race/ethnicity, and genetics account for the remaining 60% to 80%.[24] Eating disorders result in low bone density in adolescents and young adults.[25] Dieting in preadolescence and adults has been associated with reductions in bone density.[26–28]

An optimal diet with adequate intake of calcium and vitamin D is fundamental. The Institute of Medicine (IOM) recommends a daily intake of 1000 mg per day for men aged 50 to 70 years and 1200 mg per day for women older than 50 years and men older than 70 years.[29,30] Calcium supplements are added after the typical dietary calcium intake is determined so that the total daily intake is achieved. Vitamin D is necessary for calcium absorption, bone health, muscle performance, and balance. The IOM recommends 600 to 1000 IU per day.[29,30] Many with osteoporosis will need more than the general recommendation. The safe upper limit for vitamin D intake for adults was increased to 4000 IU per day in 2010.[29,30] Vitamin D supplements should be recommended in amounts enough to bring the serum 25 (OH) vitamin D level to at least 30 ng/mL (75 nmol/L) to reduce fracture risk.[31]

Regular weight-bearing exercise along with core-strengthening exercises should be recommended to slow bone loss, improve balance, and increase muscle strength. Recommendations should be provided to avoid forward flexion, side-bending exercise, and lifting heavy objects. These activities can compress the spine, resulting in fractures. Fall prevention should be addressed related to environmental factors, impaired vision and hearing, medications, and some neurologic disorders affecting balance.

Counseling regarding tobacco cessation and avoiding excessive alcohol intake, if appropriate, is part of the care regimen.

Osteoporosis prescriptive treatments can significantly decrease a person's risk of experiencing a fracture. It is important to treat based on fracture risk in addition to BMD. Currently, the pharmacotherapies approved for the treatment and prevention of osteoporosis are antiresorptive or anabolic agents. The antiresorptive agents inhibit the action of osteoclasts and the anabolic agents stimulate osteoblasts to promote bone formation. Pharmacologic treatment should be initiated in the following[14,15]:

Table 3
Summary of evidence for fracture risk reduction based on drug and fracture site

Drug	Vertebral	Nonvertebral	Hip
Abaloparatide	Yes	Yes	No significant effect
Alendronate	Yes	Yes	Yes
Calcitonin	Yes	No significant effect	No significant effect
Denosumab	Yes	Yes	Yes
Ibandronate	Yes	Yes	No significant effect
Raloxifene	Yes	No significant effect	No significant effect
Risedronate	Yes	Yes	Yes
Romosozumab	Yes	No significant effect	No significant effect
Teriparatide	Yes	Yes	No significant effect
Zolendronic acid	Yes	Yes	Yes

Adapted from Camacho PM, Petak SM, Binkley N, et al. American Association of Clinical Endocrinologists and American College of Endocrinology clinical practice guidelines for the diagnosis and treatment of postmenopausal osteoporosis. Endocr Pract 2016;22(suppl 4):1-42; and *Data from* Bone HG, Cosman F, Miller PD, et al. ACTIVExtend: 24 months of alendronate after 18 months of abaloparatide or placebo for postmenopausal osteoporosis. J Clin Endocrinol Metab 2018;103(8):2949-57 and Saag KG, Peterson J, Brandi ML, et al. Romosozumab or alendronate for fracture prevention in women with osteoporosis. N Engl J Med 2017;377(15):1417-27.

- Those with hip or vertebral (clinical or asymptomatic) fractures
- Those with *t*-scores ≤ -2.5 at the femoral neck, total hip, or lumbar spine by DXA
- Postmenopausal women and men age 50 and older with low bone mass (osteopenia) at the femoral neck, total hip, or lumbar spine by DXA and a 10-year hip fracture probability $\geq 3\%$ or a 10-year major osteoporosis-related fracture probability $\geq 20\%$ based on the US-adapted WHO absolute fracture risk model (FRAX)
- Selected individuals without low bone mass but high fracture risk due to risk states such as use of glucocorticoids

In addition, the American Association of Clinical Endocrinologists and American College of Endocrinology provide a treatment algorithm to guide selection of pharmacotherapy.[14] All agents have been shown to reduce the risk of vertebral fracture. Some of these have been shown also to reduce the risk of nonvertebral fractures, in some cases including hip fracture. See **Table 3** for a summary of evidence for fracture risk reduction based on drug and fracture site. There is a 30% to 87% reduction in the risk of vertebral fractures and a 16% to 25% reduction in the risk of nonvertebral fractures with pharmacologic treatment.[32–35] Fracture risk reduction can occur only with prescription adherence and persistence. Low adherence to osteoporosis pharmacotherapies has been documented since bisphosphonates first became available in 1995. Fewer than 50% of patients starting an oral bisphosphonate are still receiving this drug 1 year later.[36]

Prevention of subsequent fractures is essential. It is well documented that every fragility fracture is a sign of another impending one.[37,38] Fracture liaison services and Bone Health Management Services, coordinated by nurse practitioners, have been found to be effective in reducing subsequent fracture risk while being economical through coordinated and ongoing comprehensive patient care.[39–43]

SUMMARY

Osteoporosis is an increasing public health problem that impacts quality of life. Fractures are a common consequence of poor bone health, resulting in enormous health care, personal, and socioeconomic burden. Bone health can be managed, and osteoporosis can be prevented and diagnosed before a fracture or subsequent fracture. Nurses should consider bone health assessment and counseling as part of their standard for all patients to be forerunners in fighting this epidemic. The evidence-based information presented regarding prevention, screening, diagnosis, and treatment is intended to result in a reduction of the treatment gap and reduced fracture risk among those for whom nurses provide care.

DISCLOSURE

The author has nothing to disclose.

REFERENCES

1. Office of the Surgeon General. Bone health and osteoporosis: a report of the Surgeon General. Rockville (MD): Office of the Surgeon General; 2004.
2. NIH Consensus Development Panel on Osteoporosis Prevention, Diagnosis, and Therapy. Osteoporosis prevention, diagnosis, and therapy. JAMA 2001;285: 785–95.
3. Looker AC, Sarafrazi Isfajani N, Fan B, et al. Trends in osteoporosis and low bone mass in older US adults, 2005-2006 through 2013-2014. Osteoporos Int 2017; 28(6):1979–88.
4. Wright NC, Looker AC, Saag KG, et al. The recent prevalence of osteoporosis and low bone mass in the United States based on bone mineral density at the femoral neck or lumbar spine. J Bone Miner Res 2014;29:2520–6.
5. Burge R, Dawson-Hughes B, Solomon DH, et al. Incidence and economic burden of osteoporosis-related fractures in the United States, 2005-2025. J Bone Miner Res 2007;22:465–75.
6. Weaver J, Sajjan S, Lewiecki EM, et al. Prevalence and cost of subsequent fractures among U.S. patients with an incident fracture. J Manag Care Spec Pharm 2017;23:461–71.
7. National Committee on Quality Assurance: The state of health care quality 2014. 2014:90-91. Available at: http://www.ncqa.org/ReportCards/HealthPlans/StateofHealthCareQuality.aspx. Accessed May 24, 2019.
8. United States Bone and Joint Initiative: the burden of musculoskeletal diseases in the United States (BMUS). 4th edition. Rosemont (IL): 2019. Available at: http://www.boneandjointburden.org. Accessed May 24, 2019.
9. Agency for Healthcare Research and Quality. Medical Expenditures Panel Survey (MEPS). U.S. Department of Health and Human Services, 1998-2014. Available at: http://meps.ahrq.gov/mespweb/. Accessed May 24, 2019.
10. WHO Scientific Group. Assessment of osteoporosis at primary health care level. Summary meeting report. Brussels (Belgium): World Health Organization; 2004.
11. Melton LJ 3rd, Achenbach SJ, Atkinson EJ, et al. Long-term mortality following fractures at different skeletal sites: a population-based cohort study. Osteoporos Int 2013;24:1689–96.
12. Seeman E, Delmas PD. Bone quality – The material and structural basis of bone strength and fragility. N Engl J Med 2006;354:2250–61.
13. 2015 ISCD Official Positions – Adult. Available at: https://www.iscd.org/official-positions/2015-iscd-official-positions-adult/. Accessed May 17, 2019.
14. Camacho PM, Petak SM, Binkley N, et al. American Association of Clinical Endocrinologists and American College of Endocrinology clinical practice guidelines

for the diagnosis and treatment of postmenopausal osteoporosis. Endocr Pract 2016;22(suppl 4):1–42.

15. Cosman F, deBeur SJ, LeBoff MS, et al. Clinician's guide to prevention and treatment of osteoporosis. Osteoporos Int 2014;25:2359–81.

16. Vasikaran S, Eastell R, Bruyere O, et al. Markers of bone turnover for the prediction of fracture risk and monitoring of osteoporosis treatment: a need for international reference standards. Osteoporos Int 2011;22:391–420.

17. Siminoski K, Warshawski RS, Jen H, et al. The accuracy of historical height loss for the detection of vertebral fractures in postmenopausal women. Osteoporos Int 2006;17:290–6.

18. Tannenbaum C, Clark J, Schwartzman K, et al. Yield of laboratory testing to identify secondary contributors to osteoporosis in otherwise healthy women. J Clin Endocrinol Metab 2002;87:4431–7.

19. Kanis JA, Melton LJ, Christiansen C, et al. The diagnosis of osteoporosis. J Bone Miner Res 1994;9:1137–41.

20. Siris ES, Adler R, Bilezikian J, et al. The clinical diagnosis of osteoporosis: a position statement from the National Bone Health Alliance Working Group. Osteoporos Int 2014;25:1439–43.

21. Jamal SA, Ridout R, Chase C, et al. Bone mineral density testing and osteoporosis education improve lifestyle behaviors in premenopausal women: a prospective study. J Bone Miner Res 1999;14(12):2143–9.

22. Bunta AD, Edwards BJ, Macaulay WB Jr, et al. Own the Bone, a system-based intervention, improves osteoporosis care after fragility fractures. J Bone Joint Surg 2016;98:e109.

23. Baxter-Jones AD, Faulkner RA, Forwood MR, et al. Bone mineral accrual from 8 to 30 years of age: an estimation of peak bone mass. J Bone Miner Res 2011;26(8): 1729–39.

24. Weaver CM, Gordon CM, Janz KF, et al. The National Osteoporosis Foundation's position statement on peak bone mass development and lifestyle factors: a systematic review and implementation recommendations. Osteoporos Int 2016; 27(4):1281–386.

25. Zuckerman-Levin N, Hochberg Z, Latzer Y. Bone health in eating disorders. Obes Rev 2014;15(3):215–23.

26. Hohman EE, Balantekin KN, Birch LL, et al. Dieting is associated with reduced bone mineral accrual in a longitudinal cohort of girls. BMC Public Health 2018; 18:1285–95.

27. Bacon L, Stern JS, Keim NL, et al. Low bone mass in premenopausal chronic dieting obese women. Eur J Clin Nutr 2004;58(6):966–71.

28. Sogaard AJ, Meyer HE, Ahmed LA, et al. Does recalled dieting increase the risk of non-vertebral osteoporotic fractures? The Tromso study. Osteoporos Int 2012; 23(12):2835–45.

29. Institute of Medicine. Committee to review dietary reference intakes for vitamin D and calcium. Dietary reference intakes for calcium and vitamin D. Washington DC: National academies Press; 2011.

30. Moyer VA. Vitamin D and calcium supplementation to prevent fractures in adults: U.S. Preventive Services Task Force recommendations statement. Ann Intern Med 2013;158:691–6.

31. Bischoff-Ferrari HA, Willett WC, Wong JB, et al. Fracture prevention with vitamin D supplementation: a meta-analysis of randomized controlled trials. JAMA 2005; 293:2257–64.

32. Kanis JA, Burlet N, Cooper C, et al. European guidance for the diagnosis and management of osteoporosis in postmenopausal women. Osteoporos Int 2008; 19(4):399–428.
33. Sambrook P, Cooper C. Osteoporosis. Lancet 2006;367:2010–8.
34. Bone HG, Cosman F, Miller PD, et al. ACTIVExtend: 24 months of alendronate after 18 months of abaloparatide or placebo for postmenopausal osteoporosis. J Clin Endocrinol Metab 2018;103(8):2949–57.
35. Saag KG, Peterson J, Brandi ML, et al. Romosozumab or alendronate for fracture prevention in women with osteoporosis. N Engl J Med 2017;377(15):1417–27.
36. Curtis JR, Westfall AO, Allison JJ, et al. Channeling and adherence with alendronate and risedronate among chronic glucocorticoid users. Osteoporos Int 2006;17(8):1268–74.
37. Bliuc D, Alarkawi D, Nguyen TV, et al. Risk of subsequent fractures and mortality in elderly women and men with fragility fractures with and without osteoporotic bone density: the Dubbo Osteoporosis Epidemiology Study. J Bone Miner Res 2015;30(4):637–46.
38. Ahmed LA, Center JR, Bjornerem A, et al. Progressively increasing fracture risk with advancing age after initial incident fragility fracture: the Tromso study. J Bone Miner Res 2013;28(10):2214–21.
39. Sietsema DL, Arauju AB, Wang L, et al. The effectiveness of a private orthopaedic practice-based osteoporosis management service to reduce the risk of subsequent fractures. J Bone Joint Surg 2018;100:1819–28.
40. Walters S, Khan T, Ong T, et al. Fracture liaison services: improving outcomes for patients with osteoporosis. Clin Interv Aging 2017;12:117–27.
41. Dell R. Fracture prevention in Kaiser Permanente Southern California. Osteoporos Int 2011;22(Suppl 3):457–60.
42. Newman ED, Ayoub WT, Starkey RH, et al. Osteoporosis disease management in a rural health care population: hip fracture reduction and reduced costs in postmenopausal women after 5 years. Osteoporos Int 2003;14(2):146–51.
43. Greene D, Dell RM. Outcomes of an osteoporosis disease management program managed by nurse practitioners. J Am Acad Nurse Pract 2010;22(6):326–9.

An Update on Total Joint Arthroplasty

Current Models of Care, Strategies, and Innovations Providing the Best Patient Outcomes and the Big Changes in the Patient Experience

Adam Stephan, MSN, RN[a,b,*]

KEYWORDS

- TKA • Knee • Joint • Replacement • Surgery • Evidence based • Care models
- Outcomes

KEY POINTS

- Total knee arthroplasty numbers will continue to grow.
- Improvements in the overall processes have vastly improved.
- Patient optimization prior to surgery is key to success after surgery.
- In-patient lengths of stays are approaching 1 day or less.
- Thorough discharge education increases patient satisfaction and support patient reported outcomes.

HISTORICAL TOTAL KNEE ARTHROPLASTY

Even as few as 10 years ago, total knee arthroplasty (TKA) was a painful and exhausting surgery for the patient. With little to no preoperative education, lengthy hospital stays (>5 days), and extensive use of narcotics, it is no wonder that the average TKA patient delayed surgery until no longer able to walk without severe pain.

Once the surgery was completed and the patient was recovered, the typical TKA patient was sent to a skilled nursing facility or rehabilitation facility to 'gain strength and range of motion' prior to returning home. Infections were more common as were other complications like falls and readmissions within 30 days for a variety of reasons.

[a] HCA – Gulf Coast Division, Orthopedic Service Line; [b] National Association of Orthopaedic Nursing, Chicago, IL, USA
* National Association of Orthopaedic Nursing, 330 North Wabash Avenue, Suite 2000, Chicago, IL 60611.
E-mail address: Adam.stephan@hcahealthcare.com

Nurs Clin N Am 55 (2020) 203–208
https://doi.org/10.1016/j.cnur.2020.02.011
0029-6465/20/© 2020 Elsevier Inc. All rights reserved.

PREVALENCE OF TOTAL KNEE ARTHROPLASTY AND FUTURE PREDICTIONS

In 2018, the American Joint Replacement Registry (AJRR), the largest joint replacement database in the world, reported more than 1.1 million joint replacements completed (approximately 56% being TKA). This accounts for 25% to 30% of the estimated annual procedural volume in the United States[1] (**Fig. 1**). Primary knee replacement continues to be the number 1 elective joint replacement procedure done. As baby boomers and younger generations see the advancements in joint replacement, this number will continue to grow exponentially. According to data released from the 2018 AJRR report, the typical TKA joint replacement patient

1. Is female (58.9%)
2. Is of white race (69.5%)
3. Receives a posterior stabilized replacement with an antioxidant polyethylene liner (25 years or longer life span)
4. Is an average age of 65.5 years old[1]

All of these data imply that the typical TKA patient has a very high chance of needing only 1 replacement in a lifetime.

NURSING CARE MODEL IMPROVEMENTS

With the push for facility programs to be certified in joint replacements with an outside accrediting agency (The Joint Commission, DNV, and so forth) and to become Magnet or Malcom Baldrige certified, adaptations of traditional nursing care models for total knee replacement patients have exploded as the new standard in nursing care. Nursing care models, by the names' suggestion, are how nurses expect a typical patient to go through the system for their elective surgical process. Standardization with personalization is becoming the norm. With the typical TKA patient now having a length of stay of approximately 1 night, nursing is hard pressed to complete the same amount of education that nurses used to do in 5 days into less than 24 hours. This is where the care models have shifted the brunt of education to the patient prior to surgery.

Patient and coach education prior to surgery was validated by a study conducted by Gallup in 2015[2], proving beyond any shadow of a doubt that the only way for a patient to feel adequately prepared for elective joint replacement surgery is to have access to preoperative education.[2] Today, many facilities actually mandate that patients attend

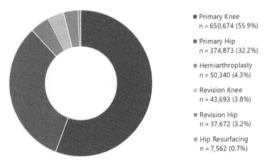

■ Primary Knee
n = 650,674 (55.9%)

■ Primary Hip
n = 374,873 (32.2%)

▪ Hemiarthroplasty
n = 50,340 (4.3%)

▫ Revision Knee
n = 43,693 (3.8%)

■ Revision Hip
n = 37,672 (3.2%)

▪ Hip Resurfacing
n = 7,562 (0.7%)

Fig. 1. A 2018 AJRR surgery run down. (*From* American Joint Replacement Registry 2018 Annual Report Figures Presentation. American Joint Replacement Registry (AJRR), 2018. Retrieved from https://ajrr.net/publications-data.)

a preoperative education class and are encouraged to bring someone who will be with them immediately after surgery.

The coach, or patient's helper, during the process of surgery is a great help. Patients are highly encouraged to bring their coaches to the preoperative class. The coaches are highly encouraged to be present as the patient is working with the health care team so a second set of eyes and ears can learn the vast information the patient is given. Coaches to the patients do not need to reside with the patient; rather, they just need to be available via telephone. The coach(es) for the patient cheerleader, chauffer, cook, and errand runner, as needed. This patient dependency phase is now reduced to a period of approximately only a week.

BEST PRACTICES THROUGH THE CONTINUUM—PATIENT OPTIMIZATION BEFORE SURGERY

Another improvement een is the use of evidence-based best practice. To achieve the best possible patient outcomes, specialty organizations and certifying agencies highly recommend the use of evidence-based best practice. Looking to the American Academy of Orthopaedic Surgeons (AAOS) and the National Association for Orthopaedic Nurses, there is a vast collection of specific clinical practice guidelines for facilities to implement in the patient's best interest. Care provided just 5 years ago for patients could now be out of date and no longer considered best practice. Best practice is an evolving science that needs constant review of current literature and research and vigilance to stay on top of the emerging data. One such area is the use of continuous passive motion devices (CPMs), a relic of prior wisdom and, in some facilities, a sacred cow.

Your mom's first TKA 15 years ago had the CPM as a gold standard; the machine was started in the hospital and then sent home to be used for anywhere from 2 weeks to a month, depending on the surgeon (**Fig. 2**). In the past decade, however, myriad evidence suggests no benefit for the standardized use of the CPM. There is research demonstrating that getting a patient up and ambulating the day of surgery is in the patient's best interest. There are facilities that are even pushing the envelope by having the patient walk from the hallway to their bed. Certifying agencies no longer will certify a joint replacement program if CPMs are in use, due to the available research showing no benefit. Evidence and recommendations for ending the use of CPM can be found in the AAOS OrthoGuidelines: http://www.orthoguidelines.org/.

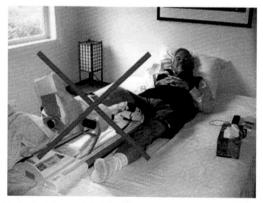

Fig. 2. The CPM. (*Adapted from* "Continuous passive motion machine" by nordique is licensed under CC BY 2.0.)

Other venues for patient presurgery optimization include universal decolonization of methicillin-resistant *Staphylococcus aureus*/methicillin-sensitive *Staphylococcus aureus*, nutritional education and the use of immunonutritional supplemental shakes, and the implementation of hard stops. Hard stop are limits set on certain criteria that serve to postpone surgery until a patient is in the acceptable criteria range. Such hard stops include the following: hemoglobin A_{1c} in diabetics must be less than 7.0 mg/dL; patients must be nonsmokers; and patients must have a body mass index less than 35 kg/m^2 - 40 kg/m^2, to name a few of the more common indices. There also has been an adaptation of the enhanced recovery after surgery (ERAS) protocol for joint replacements.[3]

IMPACT ON PATIENT OUTCOMES AND THE PATIENT EXPERIENCE

The changes in how surgery is done (robotics, better instrumentation, and so forth), the changes in preoperative patient education, and the changes in the care models all have led to improved patient-reported outcomes. **Fig. 3** best encapsulates the new model.[3]

Robotic-guided surgery is becoming more prevalent and, in the hands of a skilled robotic joint replacement surgeon, a patient may be discharged on the day of surgery. Robotic guidance can minimize incision length, minimize the amount of bone removed, and remove the guesswork from joint range-of-motion compliance; increased accuracy and precision, less soft tissue damage and injury, and increased patient satisfaction in the end result.[4]

The outcomes most monitored now, especially for certification, are preoperative education completed, use of regional anesthesia instead of general anesthesia,

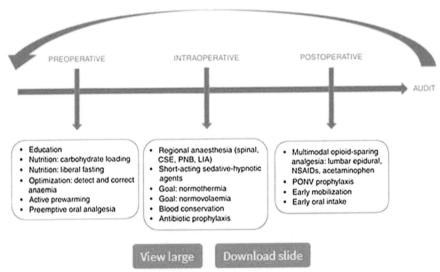

View large   Download slide

Fig. 3. ERAS protocol. A recommended protocol for ERAS for total joint arthroplasty. This diagram highlights the multimodal, multidisciplinary nature of ERAS protocol. Audit is required and is a key driver of continuous evaluation and refining of the components of care. CSE, combined spinal-epidural; ERAS, enhanced recovery after surgery; LIA, local infiltration anaesthesia; NSAID, nonsteroidal anti-inflammatory; PNB, peripheral nerve block; PONV, postoperative nausea and vomiting. (*From* E.M. Soffin, YaDeau, JT. Enhanced recovery after surgery for primary hip and knee arthroplasty: a review of the evidence. British Journal of Anesthesia. V117, issue 3 pp iii62-iii72. https://doi.org/10.1093/bja/aew362.)

ambulation of the patient day of surgery, surgical site infection rates, complication rates, discharge disposition being home (rarely using skilled nursing/rehabilitation facility), and, recently added, the patient sent home on narcotic pain medication.

RECOVERY AFTER DISCHARGE

Discharge for the TKA patient today is vastly different from just a decade ago. In today's TKA discharge world, the patient needs to have clear and conscious goals to meet prior to discharge. In the authors' facilities (HCA Gulf Coast Division, Houston, TX), a board developed by the staff is used to keep the patient, and all of the health care team, in the loop on their progress and meeting standardized goals, indicating that discharge is safe for the patient. Use of this process has tremendously increased patients' acceptance and willingness to return home with confidence.

Home recovery often is augmented with the use of outpatient physical therapy and home exercises taught by physical therapy and nursing while in the hospital. With a combination of the before mentioned items and cheering on from the coach, patients continue to improve their range of motion. Specific discharge instructions, with realistic expectations emphasized, all aid in a patient's rapid recovery. Patients no longer are expected to be bedbound or chairbound but to move and be active at least every hour or so. Expectations for recovery are laid out with calculated precision, and resources for the patient are provided. Many tools are now electronic as well, such as tracking progress via e-mail, special phone apps, or virtual therapist using video applications. An example of this can be found at AAOS OrthoInfo: https://orthoinfo. aaos.org/en/recovery/activities-after-knee-replacement/.

SUMMARY

Today's advances made in the TKA elective surgery would make mom very mad that she was unable to wait until now to have surgery. The focus has changed to creating a well-prepared patient who knows what is expected after surgery. Surgeons, anesthesiologists, and highly skilled personnel in multimodal postoperative pain optimization with regional blocks and presurgical medications replace the use of general anesthesia, removing all of the side effects and complications from yesteryear. A finely tuned health care team focused solely on a patient's recovery, who continues to reinforce the meaningful education through the discharge process, is essential. Although all the improvements made to date are eye-opening and patient-beneficial, more improvement is on the near horizon, with developments in the actual implants and materials used. Patients today can look forward to improved pain control measures, ambulating from the recovery room, and in appropriate patients, possibly eliminating the need to stay overnight in the hospital.

Mom would be so jealous if you need a TKA today!

DISCLOSURE

The author has nothing to disclose.

REFERENCES

1. American Joint Replacement Registry 2018 Annual Report Figures Presentation. American Joint Replacement Registry (AJRR) 2018. Available at: https://ajrr.net/ publications-data. Accessed September 17, 2019.

2. Ellrich M, Yu D. The benefits of pre-surgery education. GALLUP Business Journal 2015. Available at: https://news.gallup.com/businessjournal/183317/benefits-pre-surgery-education.aspx. Accessed May 20, 2015.

3. Soffin EM, YaDeau JT. Enhanced recovery after surgery for primary hip and knee arthroplasty: a review of the evidence. Br J Anesth 2016;117(3):iii62–72.

4. Khlopas A, Sodhi N, Sultan AA, et al. Robotic arm–assisted total knee arthroplasty. J Arthroplasty 2018;33(7):2002–6. Available at: https://www.clinicalkey.com/#!/content/playContent/1-s2.0-S0883540318300986?returnurl=null&referrer=null&scrollTo=%23hl0000184.

Legal Implications in the Care of Orthopedic Patients
Serious Complications

Barbara J. Levin, BSN, RN, ONC, CMSRN, LNCC[a,b,c,d,*],
Patricia Iyer, MSN, RN, LNCC[c,e]

KEYWORDS

- Complications • Cauda equina syndrome • Hematoma • Venous thrombosis
- Pulmonary embolism • Legal aspects of nursing • Standard of care

KEY POINTS

- Orthopedic nurses play a key role in adhering to the standards of care, which are defined as what a reasonably prudent nurse would do in the same or similar situation.
- Cervical spine complications are manifested by changes in breathing, swallowing, behavior (agitation or anxiety), and voice.
- Venous thromboembolism and pulmonary embolism are potentially deadly complications that may be averted by careful analysis of risk factors and prompt intervention when symptoms appear.
- Once a patient decides to sue his or her health care providers, the legal process focuses on screening the case for merit to see if it meets the 4 elements of negligence.

INTRODUCTION

Orthopedic admissions have been increasing exponentially with rising numbers of elective procedures. According to the American Academy of Orthopedic Surgeons (AAOS), there is an increase in the patient population seeking emergency orthopedic care. This increase includes patients with trauma, back pain, broken bones, sprains, and infections.[1]

There are more than 1 million total joint arthroplasties performed in the United States annually, and this number is expected to increase to nearly 4 million by 2030.[2]

Orthopedic complications can be devastating. Timely recognition and identification of a change in assessment can alter the course of care, and treatment and may be lifesaving.

[a] Clinical Scholar Orthopaedic Trauma Unit, Massachusetts General Hospital, Boston, MA, USA; [b] National Association of Orthopedic Nurses, Chicago, IL, USA; [c] American Association of Legal Nurse Consultants, Chicago, IL, USA; [d] Massachusetts Board of Registration in Nursing, Boston, MA, USA; [e] The Pat Iyer Group, 11205 Sparkleberry Drive, Fort Myers, FL 33913, USA
* Corresponding author. 8 Country Drive, Hingham, MA 02043.
E-mail address: Barbara@BarbaraJLevin.com

Nurs Clin N Am 55 (2020) 209–224
https://doi.org/10.1016/j.cnur.2020.02.003
0029-6465/20/© 2020 Elsevier Inc. All rights reserved.
nursing.theclinics.com

This article discusses the clinical signs and symptoms of 3 orthopedic complications. Case studies emphasize the clinical aspects and legal implications.

Nurses have the responsibility of providing nursing care that adheres to the standard of care. Standards of nursing care are legally defined as what a reasonably prudent nurse would do in the same or similar situation and "describe a competent level of nursing care as demonstrated by the nursing process involving assessment, diagnosis, outcome identification, planning, implementation and evaluation."[3,4]

Adverse events and resulting complications may have personal and economic consequences and affect the patient's quality of life. Orthopedic nurses play a vital role in the promotion and use of evidence-based interventions to decrease the incidence of these adverse events and improve the quality of care.[5]

NEUROVASCULAR ASSESSMENTS

Nurses must be educated on the vital role they play in performing and documenting critical neurovascular assessments. Knowledgeable nurses are empowered to provide the care expected, while maintaining patient safety. Neurovascular assessments are the hallmark of the orthopedic nursing practice. The failure to perform an adequate neurovascular assessment can result in devastating injuries, causing delay in recognition of a complication.[6] Assessments of all extremities are performed to evaluate sensory and motor function and peripheral circulation.[7]

A neurovascular assessment encompasses several components:

Color: What is the extremity color – pink, white, gray, or black? What is the capillary refill time? The ideal capillary refill is less than 3 seconds. It is measured by the time it takes for color to be restored to a nailbed after pressing on it, then releasing the pressure.

Sensation: Does the extremity have intact sensation? Are there any areas with decreased sensation?

Movement: Is the patient able to lift or move the extremity? Can the patient plantarflex (depress the foot as though pressing on the gas pedal) and dorsiflex the foot (move the foot upwards toward the head)?

Temperature: Is the extremity warm, cool or cold?

Swelling: Is swelling noted in the extremity? Compare the affected extremity and monitor any changes.

Pulse: Is pulse strong, diminished or absent? Intensity is graded on a numeric scale. 0 = absent, unable to palpate; 1+ = diminished, weaker than expected; 2+ = brisk, expected (normal); 3+ = bounding. Compare pulses from one extremity to another and monitor any changes. Report these changes immediately to the health care provider and make a new plan of care.

Pain: Extreme pain can be associated with a neurovascular deficiency. Pain with passive motion is a significant subjective complaint. This must be monitored to determine if the patient requires increasing doses of narcotics/pain medications to help with the pain.[8,9]

The nurse determines a patient's baseline and compares the affected extremity to the unaffected extremity. Performing these assessments at the beginning of care allows the nurse to determine if there are any changes noted from the previous assessments and documentation. These assessments should be documented within the medical record.

SPINE COMPLICATIONS

All patients with spine disorders are evaluated for neurologic impairment, including numbness, pain, motor function, spasm, and bowel and bladder symptoms.[6]

CERVICAL SPINE COMPLICATIONS

Common postoperative complaints may include a sore throat and surgical site pain. When assessments reveal potential complications, the nurse communicates the findings to the health care provider and makes a new plan of care to determine the cause of the symptoms and treatment needed.

Case Scenario

Patient A was a 42-year-old man with a history of weakness in his biceps and sensory loss at C6-7. His surgeon, Dr. S, recommended an anterior cervical discectomy and fusion (ACDF) C5-6, C6-7. Surgery ended at 1600, and Patient A spent an hour in the postanesthesia care unit (PACU) before his transfer to the postoperative medical surgical unit at 1700.

Patient A complained of a sore throat and neck pain. His nurse, Nurse F, medicated him with diazepam orally at 1744 and morphine intravenously at 1808. As the evening progressed, he complained of increasing pain and developed a nonproductive cough, which got louder. His voice changed from raspy to whispery. Patient A complained he "can't breathe."

Concerned about her husband, Mrs. Patient A asked Nurse F at 2015 to contact a physician to see her husband. The nurse did not act on this request and did not check on the patient until 2110, nearly an hour later.

Nurse F documented at 2120 the patient was coughing hard and felt like he was choking to death. She gave him morphine intravenously. When she offered Patient A another diazepam pill, he told her he was having difficulty breathing and could not swallow. Patient A began drooling a small amount of saliva, and his cough intensified.

At 2240, Patient A sat upright in bed, complaining of soreness and pain in his upper back. An hour later, Patient A coughed up blood. Patient A continued complaining of a sore throat, difficulty breathing, and shortness of breath. His oxygen saturation results remained normal.

Dr. S arrived at 2350, while making rounds, and ordered a stat computed tomography (CT) scan of the neck and lorazepam 1 mg intravenous push for agitation caused by coughing.

Nurse F explained to the patient and his wife that all his symptoms were normal, because her father had the same surgery and had the same symptoms.

The transport aide, unaccompanied by the nurse, brought Patient A to CT scan. Upon arrival to CT scan, Patient A stood from the wheelchair and began aggressively coughing. Patient A grabbed his neck and stopped breathing. Multiple unsuccessful attempts to intubate Patient A occurred; Patient A died in the CT scan suite.

Autopsy results determined that Patient A died as the result of an acute upper airway obstruction caused by an occlusive intraluminal laryngeal thrombus with extensive soft tissue bleeding. The extent and nature of the cervical bleed exerted a compressive force on the laryngeal tracheal structures, suffocating him (**Box 1**).

Case Analysis

There were many clinical errors that caused this catastrophic outcome. Patient A displayed signs of cervical spine complications, including

- Sore throat
- Difficulty swallowing and painful swallowing
- Difficulty managing secretions and drooling
- Difficulty breathing
- Coughing oral secretions or blood

Box 1
Cervical spine complications

Sore throat	
Difficulty swallowing/painful swallowing	
Difficulty managing secretions/drooling	
Excessive secretions	
Swelling	
Respiratory – rate, rhythm, depth	
Difficulty breathing - dyspnea	
Coughing (oral secretions or blood) – "choking to death"	May be due to aspirating on oral secretions
Breath sounds – crackles rhonchi, wheezes	
Hypoxic/cyanosis	Reduction of oxygen saturations is a late sign of airway obstruction
Stridor	Abnormal high pitched sound by a partially obstructed airway. This can be caused from airway edema
Nasal flaring	
Numbness/tingling/paralysis	
Agitation/anxiety/lethargy	
Feeling of doom	
Change in voice – hoarse voice, raspy, whispery, no voice	Phonation can change with upper airway obstruction

---

- Feeling like he was choking to death
- Agitation
- Anxiety
- Change in voice – hoarse, raspy, whispery

This case is considered a failure to rescue, which describes the outcome when a patient's condition deteriorates before the changes are recognized and acted upon. Failure to rescue is a major cause of mortality in acute care settings. Patients can display signs and symptoms of impending arrest as early as 72 hours prior to the arrest.

Nurse F failed to listen to the patient and perform assessments. Although she documented the breath sounds were clear, she testified she never listened to Patient A's breath sounds. Unfortunately, Nurse F failed to recognize the changes in Patient A's clinical presentation and falsely believed his good oxygen saturations meant he was safe. A reduction of oxygen saturations is a late sign of an airway obstruction. The nurse must treat the patient and not just rely on the numbers. Nurses cannot dismiss the clinical picture. Nurse F did not appreciate the severity of the symptoms and sent Patient A with a transport aide to CT scan when she should have traveled with him.

The deviations from the standard of care included

- Failure to recognize clinical deterioration
- Failure to communicate and escalate concerns
- Failure to physically assess the patient
- Failure to make a nursing diagnosis and treat appropriately

Cervical swelling occurs for a variety of reasons, including bleeding (hematoma). Viewing a patient's neck may reveal a subtle swollen area (**Fig. 1**). The swelling and bleeding may occur deep in the neck and be a late sign of the impending clinical catastrophe. Health care providers will not necessarily see a golf ball-size hematoma (**Fig. 2**).

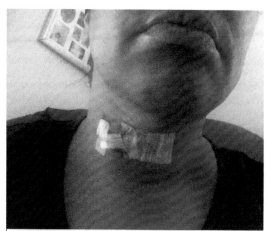

10 MINUTES AFTER THIS PHOTO WAS TAKEN,
THE PATIENT DIED OF A COMPRESSED
TRACHEA

Fig. 1. An example of swelling of the neck.

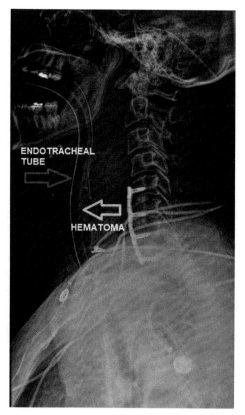

Fig. 2. Cervical hematoma.

Lessons learned from this case include the importance of listening to the patient, recognizing the change in symptoms, and being a patient advocate.

LOWER SPINE COMPLICATIONS, INCLUDING CAUDA EQUINA SYNDROME

There are a variety of postoperative lower spine complications, including swelling and hematomas. Patients may present with increased pain and/or changes in the neurovascular assessment. In addition, the patient may experience bowel or bladder difficulties.

Cauda equina syndrome is a rare disorder affecting the bundle of nerve roots (cauda equina) at the lower end of the spinal cord and is a surgical emergency. If these patients do not receive emergent attention, permanent paralysis, impaired bowel or bladder control, and loss of sexual sensation can result.[6]

Symptoms of cauda equina syndrome include

- Bowel and/or bladder dysfunction
- Severe progressive changes with lower extremities, including loss or altered sensation between the legs, over the buttocks, the inner thighs, and back of the legs (saddle area), area around the rectum, and feet/heels
- Pain, numbness or weakness spreading to one or both legs
- Suspected spinal cord compression[6]

VENOUS THROMBOEMBOLISM/PULMONARY EMBOLISM

Orthopedic procedures, especially trauma and total joint arthroplasty, place patients at an increased risk for venous thromboembolism (VTE) from the time of an injury or surgery and extend through the recovery period. "The annual number of deaths in the United States thought to be directly attributed to VTE is estimated to be 600,000 with pulmonary embolism (PE) being considered the most common preventable cause of hospital-related death. Evidence shows that VTE will occur in 3%-5% of orthopedic trauma patients despite appropriate prophylaxis."[10–12] "Despite this data, VTE has been recognized as a 'Never Event' in the eyes of Medicare payers."[10,11]

An acute PE is a form of a venous thromboembolism that is sometimes fatal. A PE originates elsewhere in the body and results in an obstruction of a pulmonary artery or one of its branches.

The evaluation of a patient with suspected deep vein thrombosis (DVT) or PE should be thorough. This enables timely diagnosis and treatment to reduce the associated morbidity and mortality and substantial health care burden. Identification of the risks and initiation of appropriate interventions to prevent or minimize complications are important roles for the nurse.

In the postoperative period, VTE is one of the most potentially life-threatening complications experienced following hip or knee arthroplasty. VTE can result in DVT that is symptomatic or asymptomatic or PE, which increases the incidence of fatal outcome.[5]

VTE is estimated to occur in approximately 35% of postoperative patients when prophylaxis is not provided.[13] Because of a high incidence in this patient population, there is broad support for VTE prophylaxis to decrease patient morbidity and mortality.[14]

The primary risk factors for VTE are patient-related, procedure-related, and anesthesia-related. "The reported incidence of DVT after a total knee replacement without prophylaxis ranges from 40 to 88%"[12] (**Box 2**).

Immobility contributes to DVT, which can lead to PEs. The optimal preventative regimen to prevent DVT after orthopedic surgery remains controversial, yet there is

Box 2
Risk factors for venous thromboembolism

Patient Related

- Older age
- Previous thromboembolism
- Malignancy
- Varicose veins
- Obesity
- Trauma
- Congestive heart failure
- Stroke
- Oral contraceptive use
- Pregnancy
- Hormone replacement therapy
- Tamoxifen therapy
- Malignancy
- Sickle cell disease
- Dehydration
- Polycythemia rubra vera
- Lupus anticoagulant
- Nephrotic syndrome
- Inflammatory bowel disease
- Intravenous drug abuse
- Deficiencies in clotting cascade related to: antithrombin III, protein C, protein S, fibrinogen, or plasminogen
- Postoperative complications: bleeding, myocardial infarction, pneumonia, urinary tract infection

Procedure Related

- Pelvic, hip, or leg surgery
- Repair of fractured pelvis or hip
- Surgery longer than 30 minutes
- Postoperative immobilization
- Postoperative infection
- Reoperation
- Intravenous therapy

Anesthesia Related

- General anesthesia

Data from Levin, B. and Cupec, P. "Complications Associated with Orthopaedic Surgeries." An Introduction to Orthopaedic Nursing, 5th Edition. NAON 2018. and Morris, N. and Levin, B. "Complications." Core Curriculum for Orthopaedic Nursing, 6th Edition. NAON 2007.

a universal consensus that some form of thromboembolic prophylaxis, especially after joint replacement, is essential.[10,15]

Many facilities collect thromboembolism risk data to help identify patients who have a low, moderate or high risk for VTE. Oftentimes these assessments use an algorithm to guide prevention depending on the identified risk level. All nurses should be aware of the risk factors to help identify patients at high risk and implement preventative measures.

Anticoagulation remains the cornerstone of prevention and treatment for VTE. Currently there are a variety of anticoagulation agents, including unfractionated low-dose heparin, low molecular-weight heparin, Factor Xa Inhibitors such as rivaroxaban (Xarelto) and apixaban (Eliquis), Warfarin (Coumadin), fondaparinux (Arixtra), vitamin K antagonists (VKA) and antiplatelet therapy (Clopidrogel/Plavix), and aspirin.

The combination of both chemical and non-pharmacologic prophylaxis has been shown to have a greater therapeutic effect than either modality alone.[10]

Nonpharmacological interventions include:

- Promote early ambulation
- Use graduated elastic stockings to reduce venous hypertension, decrease edema, and improve microcirculation
- Avoid stockings that are too tight as they increase venous pressure below the knee and delay venous emptying
- Apply intermittent pneumatic compression devices
- Supply a foot impulse pump
- Instruct in frequent plantarflexion and dorsiflexion of the foot, ankle, and toes
- Teach deep breathing exercises to help the large veins empty by increasing negative pressure in the thorax
- Keep the patient well hydrated
- Use bone vacuum technique during surgery
- Insert inferior vena cava filters[5,16]

"Inferior Vena Cava Filters may be beneficial in trauma patients at high risk for PE (spinal cord injury, head injury with Glasgow Coma Score <8 for more than 48 hours, older than 55 years with lower extremity fracture, and pelvic fracture with associated long-bone fracture) and who cannot be anticoagulated."[10]

A PE has various presenting clinical features. The most common symptoms are tachycardia, dyspnea, and low oxygen saturation.[17] The clinical presentation can be notoriously unreliable, as many embolisms are silent[17] (**Box 3**). "The current gold standard diagnostic instruments are venography for deep vein thrombosis and pulmonary angiography for pulmonary embolism. However, because these tests are invasive and expensive, alternative diagnostic tools include venous compression ultrasonography for deep vein thrombosis and ventilation-perfusion scans and computed tomographic pulmonary angiogram for pulmonary embolism"[18] (**Figs. 3** and **4**).

Case Scenario

Patient B was a 37-year-old teacher admitted to the hospital after sustaining a fall while playing basketball with her students. She was diagnosed with a right comminuted tibial plateau fracture. She took amlodipine for hypertension, was 5 feet 3 inches tall and weighed 167 pounds. In the operating room, Dr. L, the orthopedic surgeon, applied a right leg external fixator as part of a closed reduction. Because of her pain and immobility, Patient B required a full hospital admission.

Nurse G completed the admission assessment, which included a venous thrombosis risk assessment. The nurse incorrectly completed the form. Nurse G missed

Box 3
Physical examination of patients with pulmonary embolism

Neurologic

Apprehensive

Restlessness

Confusion

Anxiety

Lightheadedness

Respiratory

Dyspnea

Cough

Hemoptysis

Abnormal respiratory rate/pattern

Decreased breath sounds

Abnormal breath sounds (crackles, wheezes)

Hypoxia

Tachypnea

Cyanosis

Cardiac

Tachycardia

Palpitations

Split S2

Abnormal blood pressure (hypotension)

Syncope

Chest pain

Vascular

Distended neck veins

Positive hepatojugular reflex

Integumentary

Cool or warm skin temperature

Diaphoresis

Pallor, cyanosis, sluggish capillary refill

Fever

Leg pain (Homan sign). although not specific or sensitive to DVT and present in less than one-third of symptomatic patients.

Data from Morris, N. and Levin, B. "Complications." Core Curriculum for Orthopaedic Nursing, 6th Edition. Page 187. NAON 2007.

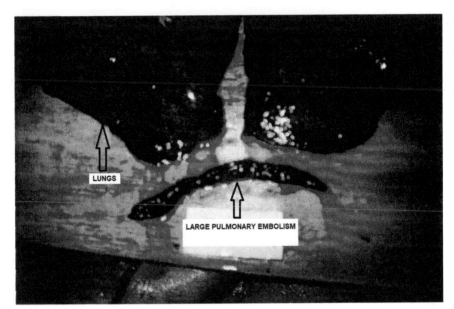

Fig. 3. Pulmonary embolism.

scoring "leg fracture," and later in the admission, the nursing staff did not consider her prolonged bedrest as increasing her risk for venous thrombosis. This would have added 2 additional points to give a score of 7 (**Fig. 5**). A score of 5 or more categorizes a patient at the highest risk for DVT according to this hospital's policy.

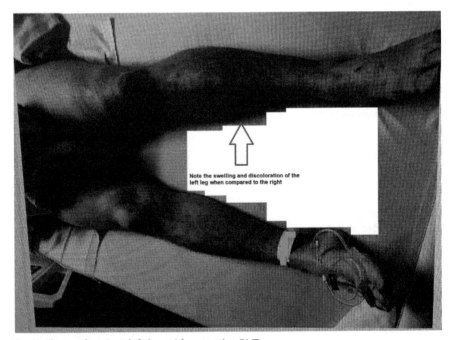

Fig. 4. Photo of patient left leg with extensive DVT.

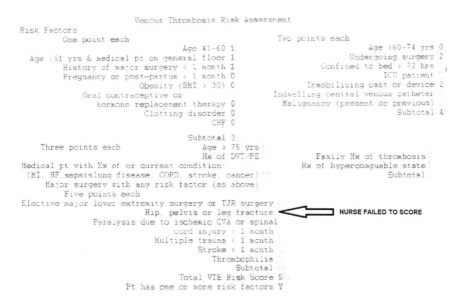

Venous Thrombosis Risk Assessment

Risk Factors

One point each
Age 41-60 1
Age <61 yrs & medical pt on general floor 1
History of major surgery < 1 month 1
Pregnancy or post-partum < 1 month 0
Obesity (BMI > 30) 0
Oral contraceptive or
hormone replacement therapy 0
Clotting disorder 0
CHF 0

Subtotal 3

Two points each
Age >60-74 yrs 0
Undergoing surgery 2
Confined to bed > 72 hrs
ICU patient
Immobilizing cast or device 2
Indwelling central venous catheter
Malignancy (present or previous)
Subtotal 4

Three points each
Age > 75 yrs
Hx of DVT/PE
Medical pt with Hx of or current condition:
(MI, HF, sepsis lung disease, COPD, stroke, cancer)
Major surgery with any risk factor (as above)
Family Hx of thrombosis
Hx of hypercoaguable state
Subtotal

Five points each
Elective major lower extremity surgery or TJR surgery
Hip, pelvis or leg fracture   ⟵ NURSE FAILED TO SCORE
Paralysis due to ischemic CVA or spinal
cord injury < 1 month
Multiple trauma < 1 month
Stroke < 1 month
Thrombophilia
Subtotal
Total VTE Risk Score 5
Pt has one or more risk factors Y

Fig. 5. Risk for DVT scale.

Postoperative day #1
The physical therapist evaluated Patient B while she was having severe right leg pain. Patient B was able to stand at the bedside with maximum assistance. Patient B was not out of bed for the remainder of the shift. She complained of difficulties moving her right leg in bed.

Postoperative day #2
Patient B required maximum assistance to roll side to side and to sit at the bedside. She complained of 10/10 pain and was unable to stand at the bedside with the physical therapist. Dr. L documented, "Patient seen and examined and doing well, pain controlled. Calf soft compressible. May be discharged home." Dr. M (the hospitalist) documented "DVT prophylaxis," yet Patient B was neither on DVT prophylaxis medications nor on any nonpharmacologic measures.

Postoperative day #3
Patient B's nurse observed the patient had right leg edema when he assisted her out of bed with 2-person maximum assistance to sit in a chair for 30 minutes. Patient B was unable to walk and could not plantarflex or dorsiflex, which she had previously been able to do.

Patient B complained of muscle spasms and pain in her right lower extremity, left rib cage, and upper abdomen. Her heart rate was 125 at rest; her blood pressure was 106/86. None of this information was communicated to the orthopedic surgeon.

Postoperative day #4
Dr. M documented, "Patient B is here with inability to ambulate status post right tibial plateau fracture with non-weight bearing on the right lower extremity." Dr. M requested Patient B be out of bed as tolerated. Dr. M documented: "Deep venous thrombosis prophylaxis – this patient currently is not receiving – would consider adding subcutaneous Heparin versus aspirin, dependent on the risk assessment per

orthopedic surgery." Given the patient was scheduled to have an open reduction internal fixation surgery within the next 2 weeks, once the leg swelling decreased, Dr. M recommended she have inpatient rehabilitation due to her trouble walking.

Patient B was able to stand and ambulate five feet with moderate assistance. The physical therapist noted Patient B's anxiety level was 7 to 8/10; she complained of fatigue as well as muscle spasms in the right lower extremity upon movement. She sat up for about 10 minutes and returned to bed.

The occupational therapist worked with Patient B, who requested to use the commode. After a few minutes, she told her nurse, "I feel dizzy," and then she "passed out" and coded. The code team attempted resuscitation efforts for 80 minutes without success.

Case Analysis

In this tragic case, the hospital policy required the nursing staff to complete the VTE risk assessment daily. The physicians were not properly educated on the use of this tool or the order sets that went along with this assessment.

The initial physician's postoperative orders failed to address DVT prophylaxis. The nursing staff failed to score Patient B appropriately, overlooking her leg fracture. Despite the lack of this component, Patient B scored as a high risk and thus required a plan to prevent VTE. The admissions nurse and orthopedic surgeon each violated the standard of care by failing to discuss the plan of DVT prophylaxis. Dr. M indicated in her note that she would discuss the DVT prophylaxis plan with the orthopedic surgeon; she never did.

During Patient B's 4-day admission, the medical record established there was no order placed for DVT prophylaxis and specifically no order placed for a blood thinner. There were no daily VTE risk reassessments completed while Patient B remained an inpatient.

An autopsy determined Patient B's cause of death was acute PE arising out of a DVT in her right leg after external fixation of the right knee. Dr. P, the pathologist, testified the DVT likely formed the day prior to her death. She had clots in both her pulmonary veins and arteries, the latter of which probably occurred minutes prior to her death. Further, she testified the contributing factors to the formation of clots and ultimate death included blunt force trauma injury to the right leg, immobilization, surgery, obesity, and the lack of DVT prophylaxis medications.

The nursing expert witness concluded the nurses failed to properly follow the nursing process with respect to their care and treatment. The nursing staff failed to complete daily VTE risk assessments. At trial, the expert further testified Patient B was at high risk for blood clots, and because of her lack of mobility and persistent swelling of the right lower extremity, she should have been reassessed daily.

The standard of care required the nurses to communicate the changes to the physicians, which would have led to a physician order for an anticoagulant. There are well-known risk factors for blood clots that a reasonably careful nurse attending to a postoperative inpatient should recognize without consulting the hospital's VTE risk assessment. After assessing Patient B as a high risk for VTE, the next step in the nursing process was to develop a plan to protect Patient B from blood clots. The hospital protocol requires both blood thinner and sequential compression devices (SCDs), which were not used.

The nursing staff members also violated their duty to advocate for Patient B. They had a high-risk patient whom they should have known required protection from potentially fatal blood clots.

Case Scenario

Orthopedic Nurse H opened a certified letter and saw this sentence: "You are being sued by Patient C for nursing negligence." Nurse H did not remember Patient C as a patient and had no idea why she was being sued.

A lot of behind-the-scenes work occurs before a health care professional receives a notice of a lawsuit in the form of a complaint. The first step in the investigation of a potential claim occurs when a person at the law firm (legal nurse consultant, paralegal, or attorney) interviews the potential plaintiff (the person who wishes to bring the suit). Patient C experienced cauda equina syndrome. In his interview, Patient C explained to Attorney T what happened: what he was like before his spinal surgery, how he lost motor and sensation after surgery, and how his life has changed.

Patient C explained, "I want to sue the doctor and nurses who took care of me. Look at what happened to me. I can't work; the bills are mounting; we are at risk of losing our home. My wife is trying to manage everything – her job, the household chores I used to do, and the help I need. It is too much. I can't walk. I must wear diapers, just like a baby. It is demeaning."

Patient C was overwhelmed by the changes in his life. Other reasons why people seek plaintiff attorney include the desire to

- Punish the healthcare provider
- Take away the provider's license to practice
- Force the medical provider to acknowledge there was a medical error
- Receive an apology
- Obtain all the facts of what happened
- Get assurance that this will not happen again and fix the system
- Receive appropriate compensation to help with the financial stressors[19]

Some individuals who have valid medical malpractice cases do not seek an attorney. This might occur because they

- Like their health care providers
- Do not understand the process of filing a lawsuit
- Accept an apology for a mistake
- Do not realize someone made a mistake
- Believe their medical care costs will increase if they file a suit
- Are convinced no one in their geographic area will treat them if they become known as a person who sued a health care provider
- Think being injured was their fate
- Do not have the funds to invest in pursuing a claim
- Are not willing to go through the prolonged processes of a lawsuit
- Have aspects of their lives that they do not want to put under scrutiny, such as substance abuse problems

E, the legal nurse consultant (LNC), provided an opinion on the merits of Patient C's potential claim. As the LNC dug into the medical records, he found when Patient C returned from the postanesthesia care unit at 1000, Nurse H noted he could move his legs and his skin was warm to touch. This baseline assessment was critical in comparing Patient C's condition as he recovered from surgery.

The next entry at 1200 stated that Patient C complained of numbness from his feet to his hips. Nurse H documented, "Assured patient he was feeling effects of spinal anesthesia. Will monitor." At 1500, Patient C told Nurse H he was having trouble moving his legs. She again assured him what he was feeling was normal.

Change of shift took place at 1900. When Nurse H gave Nurse J (the incoming nurse) the report, she explained that Patient C had some minor numbness and movement issues because of the anesthesia, and there was nothing to be concerned about.

Nurse J made rounds at 2000, noted the patient had no feeling or movement in his legs, and documented, "Will monitor." Patient C was unable to urinate, so Nurse J obtained an order for a straight catheterization and drained 1400 cc at 2300. Nurse J monitored Patient C every 5 or 6 hours throughout the night and each time noted the absence of sensation and movement of his legs. Believing these changes were because of anesthesia, Nurse J did not notify anyone of G's condition.

At 0800 the next day, when the neurosurgeon made rounds, she was shocked to find Patient C was paralyzed. A stat MRI showed an expanding spinal epidural hematoma. Emergency surgery to drain the hematoma failed to reverse the spinal cord damage.

LEGAL ANALYSIS

LNC E considered the 4 elements of a successful medical malpractice case, knowing the value of a careful screening and the expense of litigation. These include: duty, breach of duty, injury and damages. Attorney T's law firm would spend at least $100,000 and 3 to 5 years pursuing a claim.

LNC E concluded Patient C had damages. His paralysis was permanent. He had incontinence, risks for pressure sores and urinary tract infections and other complications of immobility. LNC E knew these injuries were serious and costly.

Next, LNC E considered the duty of the 2 shifts of nurses. Each nurse assigned to Patient C was obligated to assess his postoperative condition. Nurse H and Nurse J had a duty to follow the standard of care in their actions, that of a reasonably prudent nurse in the same or similar situation. The reasonably prudent nurse would note changes in sensation and motor and report those changes to the surgeon.

LNC E concluded that although Nurse H and Nurse J obtained concerning assessment data, they breached the standard of care by not informing the surgeon of the abnormalities. This deprived the patient of the opportunity to get prompt neurosurgical attention. LNC E was confident that a neurosurgical expert witness would back up his conclusion of the nurse's failure to report Patient C's change in condition was the proximate cause of his damages (cauda equina syndrome).

As LNC E thought about the observations of the 2 nurses, he concluded, "They collected assessment data, but not frequently enough. The standard of care required them to evaluate the patient's motor and sensation every 4 hours. When they saw the changes, they should have increased the frequency of monitoring and asked the surgeon to come in to assess the patient. Their failure to use critical thinking contributed to the delay in diagnosis of the hematoma."

After LNC E provided the attorney with his analysis of the case, Attorney T filed suit, and Nurse H and Nurse J were notified they were defendants. Nurse H decided that since she did not remember Patient C, she would look at his medical record the next time she went to work. As she stared at her notes, she thought, "Surely I would have told the neurosurgeon about his numbness. I think I did. Didn't I? I could add a note that says I informed the neurosurgeon at 1500 when I discovered Patient C could not move his leg. That would make me look better."

When Nurse H added a note into the chart stating she informed the surgeon of Patient C's changes, she set in motion a cascade of events that undermined her nursing career.

Nurse H brought a copy of her altered notes to her deposition (being asked questions under oath). Attorney T asked her to go through her notes, line by line. When Nurse H testified she reported the changes to the neurosurgeon, Attorney T immediately asked her to point to that entry in the medical records.

Attorney T compared her set of medical records supplied by the hospital before she filed suit, with Nurse H's altered medical records, and in that moment, shook her head. She knew a chart audit would show when the late entry was added. The neurosurgeon had testified at her deposition that no one told her of the changes.

Nurse H's attempt to cover up her failure to report Patient C's condition is called spoliation of evidence, an intentional alteration of medical records related to pending or active litigation. There are severe consequences for such actions. The legal system recognizes that altering medical records impairs the opposing party's ability to pursue a claim. This deliberate manipulation of the records greatly increases the odds the health care provider or entity will settle the case, rather than risk angering a jury with a cover up. The greatest risk is that an angry jury would award punitive damages, which are designed to punish the health care provider involved in changing the record. Punitive damages are not covered by insurance policies and are thus paid out of pocket.

If a patient or family sues the health care team, the legal system takes over. After a careful screening of the case for merit, a lawsuit begins. A health care provider should never give in to the temptation to alter medical records. To do so is fatal to the defense of a case.

Nurse H's willful and intentional wrongdoing was reported to her state's board of nursing. After an investigation of the behavior, the board of nursing suspended Nurse H's license to practice nursing.

SUMMARY

To help reduce potentially devastating outcomes from spinal complications and venous thromboembolism, it is essential for the bedside nurse to have a comprehensive understanding of risk factors and appropriate assessments. The orthopedic nurse is a vital member of the health care team and carries a responsibility for accurately assessing, documenting, and mobilizing the team when abnormal changes occur.

It is not acceptable for nurses to be passive members of the team, with a role confined to only observing and charting. Nurses act as patient advocates rooted in their awareness of the vulnerabilities of their patients. With knowledge of the risk factors and complications associated with patients under their care, the bedside nurse must communicate with the physician. Together, they create a plan of care that includes determining the rationale for the changes in assessments and care.

DISCLOSURE

The authors have nothing to disclose.

REFERENCES

1. Emergency Orthopaedic Care. AAOS position statement 1172. Rosemont (IL): American Academy of Orthopaedic Surgeons; 2015.
2. Etkin C, Springer B. The American joint replacement registry – the first 5 years. Arthroplast Today 2017;(2):67–9.
3. Bowe P, Harrington D, Jurlano M, et al. American Nurses Association recognition of a nursing specialty, approval of a specialty nursing scope of practice

statement, acknowledgement of specialty nursing standards of practice, and affirmation of focused practice competencies. Silver Spring (MD): American Nurses Association; 2017.

4. Harvey CV, David J, Eckhouse DR, et al. The National Association of Orthopaedic Nurses (NAON) Scope and Standards of Orthopaedic Nursing Practice, Third Edition. Orthop Nurs 2013;32:139.

5. Smith MA, Walsh C, Levin B, et al. Orthopaedic snafus: when adverse events happen in orthopaedics. Orthop Nurs 2017;36(2):98–109.

6. Levin B, Mooney N. Orthopaedic nursing malpractice issues. In: Iyer P, Levin B, Ashton K, et al, editors. Nursing malpractice, 4th edition, Vol. II – Roots of nursing malpractice. Tucson (AZ): Lawyers & Judges Publishing; 2011. p. 253–78.

7. Lau B, Haut E, Maheshwari B, et al. Hospital acquired DVT/PE as 'never events': a misguided strategy for performance improvement in VTE prevention. Blood 2012; 120:3180.

8. Schreiber ML. Neurovascular assessment: an essential nursing focus. Medsurg Nurs 2016;25(1):55–7.

9. Sarauer N. Musculoskeletal Anatomy and Neurovascular Assessment. In: Zychowicz ME, editor. An introduction to orthopaedic nursing. 5th edition. Chicago (IL): NAON; 2018. p. 1–16.

10. Sagi HC, Ahn J, Ciesla D, et al. Venus thromboembolism prophylaxis in orthopaedic trauma patients: a survey of OTA member practice patterns and OTA expert panel recommendations. J Orthop Trauma 2005;29(10):E355–62.

11. Levin B, Cupec P. Complications associated with orthopaedic surgeries. In: Zychowicz ME, editor. An introduction to orthopaedic nursing. 5th edition. Chicago (IL): NAON; 2018. p. 137–63.

12. Beckman MG, Hooper WC, Critchley SE, et al. Venous thromboembolism. Am J Prev Med 2010;38(4):S495–501.

13. Mostafavi Tabatabae R, Rasouli MR, Maltenfort MG, et al. Cost effective prophylaxis against venous thromboembolism after total joint arthroplasty: warfarin v. aspirin. J Arthroplasty 2015;30:159–64.

14. Lapidus LJ, Ponzer S, Pettersson H, et al. Symptomatic venous thromboembolism and mortality in orthopaedic surgery – an observational study of 45,968 consecutive procedures. BMC Musculoskelet Disord 2013;14:177. Available at: http://www.biomedcentral.com/1471-2474/14/177.

15. Rachidi S, Aldin ES, Greenberg C, et al. The use of novel oral anticoagulants for thromboprophylaxis after elective major orthopaedic surgery. Expert Rev Hematol 2013;6(6):677–95.

16. Levin BJ, Morris NS. Complications in orthopaedics. In: Core curriculum for orthopaedic nursing. 6th edition. Chicago (IL): NAON; 2007. p. 175–208.

17. Tornetta P, Bogdan Y. Pulmonary embolism in orthopaedic patients: diagnosis and management. J Acad Orthop Surg 2012;20(9):586–95.

18. Saleh J, El-Othmani MM, Saleh KJ. Deep vein thrombosis and pulmonary embolism considerations in orthopedic surgery. Orthop Clin North Am 2017;48(2): 127–35.

19. Iyer P, Levin B, Ashton K, et al. Nursing Malpractice, 4th edition, volume 1 "foundations of nursing malpractice claims" and volume ii "roots of nursing malpractice.". Tucson (AZ): Lawyers & Judges Publishing; 2011.

Pain Management for Orthopedic Patients; Closing the Gap

Rachel Torani, MSN, MBA, BSN, RN[a],*, Debra Byrd, BSN, RN, ONC[b]

KEYWORDS

- Joint replacement • Pain • Opioid • Patient experience • Nonpharmacologic
- Multimodal • Distraction therapy

KEY POINTS

- Total joint replacement (TJR) is a common and frequent surgery performed for treatment of end-stage osteoarthritis and is one of the most painful surgeries.
- The history of pain assessment regulations shaped the current practice of orthopedic nursing.
- The opioid epidemic is requiring health care professionals to seek out alternative therapies for treatment of postoperative pain.
- Nonopioid pharmacologic and nonpharmacologic approaches to pain management have emerged to reduce the use of opioids.
- Thorough education of nurses, patients, and their caregivers on pain reduction techniques improves the pain experience.

INTRODUCTION

Total joint replacement (TJR) is the most common treatment of advanced osteoarthritis when conservative measures have failed.[1,2] The chronic and painful nature of osteoarthritis is the most common precipitating factor for individuals seeking TJR surgery.[3] TJR is extremely effective in relieving the chronic pain condition, restoring function, and improving quality of life.[4,5] Because of the effectiveness of the surgery, it is one of the most commonly performed surgeries in the United States.[5]

TJR volumes have increased over the past few decades; in a recent study by Sloan and colleagues[6] (2018), a linear regression model was used to predict future volumes through 2030 and 2060 (**Fig. 1**).[7] In the same study it was shown that the ages of the population receiving TJR surgery are decreasing in both men and women (**Table 1**). This finding is significant for the future population and health care resources that will be needed.

[a] Orthopedic Institute, AdventHealth, Orlando, FL, USA; [b] Specialty Service Lines, AdventHealth, Celebration, FL 34747, USA
* Corresponding author. Nursing Administration, 400 Celebration Place, Celebration, FL 34747.
E-mail address: Rachel.Torani@AdventHealth.com

Nurs Clin N Am 55 (2020) 225–238
https://doi.org/10.1016/j.cnur.2020.02.004
0029-6465/20/© 2020 Elsevier Inc. All rights reserved.

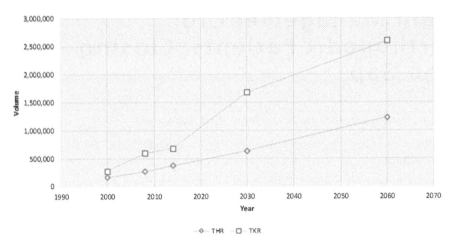

Fig. 1. TJR average volume by year; linear regression analysis. THR, total hip replacement; TJR, total joint replacement; TKR, total knee replacement. (*Data from* Sloan MMM, Premkumar A,M, Sheth N,M. Projected Volume of Primary Total Joint Arthroplasty in the U.S., 2014-2030. 0014030. 2018:1455-1460 and Newswire P. Projected volume of primary and revision total joint replacement in the U.S. 2030 to 2060. *Cision PR Newswire.* March 6, 2018. https://www.prnewswire.com/news-releases/projected-volume-of-primary-and-revision-total-joint-replacement-in-the-us-2030-to-2060-300608386.html.)

Although effective in restoring function and improving quality of life, TJR is one of the most painful surgeries performed. A study performed in Germany consisting of 105 hospitals compared pain outcomes among 30 different surgical procedures. The results of this study ranked total knee replacement and total hip replacement as 5 and 11 out of 30 respectively.[8] In addition, the literature suggests that one-third of the population receiving TJR experience moderate to severe pain in the immediate postoperative period.[9,10]

Severe pain after TJR is associated with poor outcomes (**Fig. 2**).[2,4,5,8,11]

Managing the pain experience is essential to improving these outcomes. The disparity in outcomes between severe unmanaged pain and effective pain management puts a spotlight on the need for a better understanding of the pain experience, challenges to effective pain management, and improved pain management strategies for health care professionals. Effective pain management leads to improved outcomes.[3,10,12,13] The historical practice of orthopedic nursing must evolve to meet the new paradigm.

Table 1
Mean age and incidence of total joint replacement recipients

	2000		2014	
	Mean Age (y)	Incidence	Mean Age (y)	Incidence
Male	66.3	60.65	64.9	188.15
Female	68.0	92.85	65.9	193.25

Incidence per 1000 population, average of hip and knee.
Data from Sloan MMM, Premkumar A,M, Sheth N,M. Projected Volume of Primary Total Joint Arthroplasty in the U.S., 2014-2030. 0014030. 2018:1455-1460.

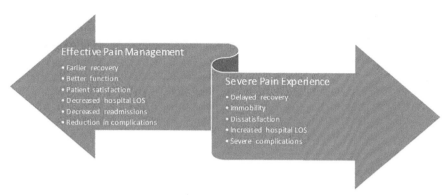

Fig. 2. Pain experience outcomes. LOS, length of stay. (*Data from* Refs.[2,4,5,8,11])

PAIN
Types of Pain

For orthopedic patients, in the simplest form, pain can be broken down into 2 categories: acute and chronic. Acute pain, as defined by the US Centers for Disease Control and Prevention (CDC), is the result of a surgery or traumatic injury and typically does not persist past 3 months.[14] Chronic pain is any pain that persists past the 3-month period.[14] The acute pain response is a physiologic response involving the sympathetic nervous system.[12] This response involves almost all body systems (**Table 2**). Chronic pain has a psychological effect. Patients with chronic pain conditions can experience anxiety, depression, relationship disfunction, feelings of helplessness, and loss of employment.[15] Patients seeking TJR surgery are often in a chronic pain state.

Predictors of Pain

To better manage the pain experience, health care providers need to understand the patient's current pain state and predictors for complex or increased risk for poor pain experience. The most common risk factors for poor pain experience in the acute

Table 2		
Physiologic response of acute pain		
	Increase	**Decrease**
Heart rate	X	—
Oxygen consumption	X	—
Blood pressure	X	—
Cardiac output	X	—
Respiratory rate	X	—
Respiratory depth	—	X
Gastrointestinal motility	—	X
Genitourinary motility	—	X
Nausea	X	—
Vomiting	X	—
Secretion of cortisol	X	—

Data from Goode V, Morgan B, Muckler V, et al. Multimodal Pain Management for Major Joint Replacement Surgery. *National Assocication of Orthopaedic Nurses.* March/April 2019;38(2):150-156.

postoperative period are young age, female gender, and chronic pain with high intensity.[1,8,15]

A study performed by Lindberg and colleagues[1] (2017) found that patients with high pain scores before surgery had a worse pain trajectory in the acute postoperative period. In addition, on the day of surgery, the more hours that a patient remained in high levels of pain the worse their long-term pain trajectory.[1] From this it can be inferred that aggressive postoperative pain management regimens improve the patients' pain experience in the acute postoperative phase. In addition, knowledge of modifiable increased pain risk factors could enable providers the ability to implement appropriate interventions to decrease the postoperative pain experience.[1]

History of Pain Assessment Regulations

In 1995, the American Pain Society and the American Society of Anesthesiologists introduced the idea of pain as the fifth vital sign; shortly after, the Joint Commission implemented new standards for assessing and reassessing pain.[16] In 2010, with the implementation of the Affordable Care Act, hospital-level accountability was solidified by tying reimbursement to the Hospital Consumer Assessment of Healthcare Providers and Systems patient satisfaction surveys.[4,11]

These laws and regulations created an environment in which opioid medications became the orthopedic surgeon's primary choice in treating pain after TJR surgery. For decades, nurses administered opioids to their patients to reduce the postoperative pain and provide a level of comfort that patients expect and need to participate in their physical therapy sessions. The current statistics defining an opioid crisis in the United States require care givers to seek alternative measures to treat postoperative pain.

Challenges to Pain Control

Adequate pain control and appropriate treatment continue to challenge orthopedic health care providers around the globe. One of these challenges is pain assessment tools. At present, the most commonly used pain assessment tools (ie, numeric pain scale, visual analog scale [VAS]) are subjective and do not contain an objective measurement of pain. Despite that fact, these tools are widely accepted and provide a universal measure for the subjective pain experience.

Another challenge to pain control is the long history of first-line treatment involving opioids.[5] Opioids come with common side effects of sedation, nausea, vomiting, dizziness, and so forth.[9] Many of these side effects are undesirable to both the patient and practitioner, affecting the immediate recovery period. In addition to the side effects, patients have a concern about becoming addicted to opioids,[11] which is a real concern in the current paradigm with the opioid epidemic.

Opioids are the most commonly prescribed analgesic medications by orthopedic surgeons, accounting for 7% of all opioids prescribed in the United States.[10] In a 2017 article published in *AARP*, "America's Addiction to Pain Pills," the hospitalization rate for individuals 65 years of age and older quintupled in the last 2 decades.[17] From the CDC, in 2016 there were 42,000 opioid deaths and, of those deaths, 40% (46/d) involved prescription drugs.[18] These staggering statistics have made the opioid epidemic a national priority. There have been laws passed by the House and Senate to establish programs for prevention, treatment, a recovery of opioids.[18] This focus has extended to the state level, with increased monitoring of prescribing and limits on the quantities of opioids that can be prescribed for acute pain.

OPIOID CRISIS EFFECT ON NURSING PRACTICE

Nurses are qualified and well positioned as frontline caregivers to support coordinated efforts to address the epidemic.[16] In the National Association of Orthopaedic Nurses (NAON) 2018 position statement on the opioid crisis, an increase in provider and patient education and the use of multimodal and alternative therapies are highly recommended.[19] The use of these therapies has proved to be an important first step in eliminating decades of opioid-focused practice. Nurses require an extensive knowledge of multimodal and alternative therapies to relay information to their patients. Proper education on multimodal and alternative therapies for all providers is a key factor in expectation modification for both the providers and the patients undergoing TJR surgery.

Mandatory preoperative education is listed at a best practice in NAON's 2018 Best Practice Guidelines to total knee replacement and total hip replacement for the patients and their caregivers.[20,21] A literature review was completed that included 25 studies addressing preoperative education. Six of those studies reported statistical significance in relation to preoperative education reducing length of stay, falls, complications, and financial charges.[22–26] Mandatory preoperative education continues to be a challenge for some orthopedic programs; it requires full participation from the facility and the orthopedic surgeons.

Preoperative education is the first step in managing the patient experience. In this course, patients and their caregivers are educated on the surgical process, exercises, prevention of complications, and so forth, and, most importantly, on pain expectations and the treatment plan. It is important to implement different learning styles, whether it is through reading, writing, visual approaches, or auditory approaches. This education ensures that patients are adequately prepared for the immediate postoperative period and the recovery at home. Patients should be made aware of the opioid epidemic and the risk of addiction along with education on how an alternative treatment plan such as multimodal and alternative therapies will decrease their need for opioids.

SOLUTIONS TO ADEQUATE PAIN CONTROL, PHARMACOLOGIC
Multimodal

The implementation of a multimodal pain management protocol has proved to be an important first step in eliminating decades of opioid-focused practice. Multimodal pain management is the use of multiple analgesic agents or techniques that have actions on different pain mechanisms to provide pain relief.[10,12] Nonopioid medications (**Table 3**) are given at different times throughout the surgical process, starting days before surgery. In the preoperative phase, these medications prevent the biochemical pain cascade before it begins by acting on specific pain receptor sites.[10] Nursing education on how each new medication targets different pain receptors and its effect on reducing the need for opioid medications is imperative to the success of a new multimodal program. Specific education around nonsteroidal antiinflammatory medications, cyclooxygenase II inhibitors, neurotransmitter inhibitors, gabapentinoids, acetaminophen, and muscle relaxers should be provided to frontline nurses. Note that there is not a specific optimal protocol or clear time frame on administration of these medications.[10,12]

In using a multimodal approach to pain management, it is important to consider the safety of the medications. There are no current risk stratification guidelines on the use of these medications, and it is up to the care delivery team to determine the safety of administration for each patient.[10] Comorbidities include (see **Table 3**):

Table 3
Common multimodal nonopioid analgesics and their effects

Modality	Medications	Mechanism of Action	Effect	Considerations
NSAIDs	Aspirin, ibuprofen, ketorolac, celecoxib, naproxen, meloxicam, diclofenac	Inhibited synthesis and release of prostaglandins and COX-2	Antiinflammatory, analgesic antipyretic	Gastrointestinal bleeding, renal injury/failure
Acetaminophen	Tylenol	Inhibited synthesis and release of prostaglandins	Analgesic, antipyretic	Hepatotoxicity
NMDA antagonists	Ketamine	NMDA antagonist	Potentiate the effect of opioids, analgesic	Increases intracranial pressure; increases blood pressure
Gabapentinoids	Neurontin, Lyrica	Alter neurotransmission in the dorsal horn of the spinal cord	Decrease neuropathic pain	Dizziness, drowsiness, confusion

Abbreviations: COX, cyclooxygenase; NMDA, *N*-methyl-D-aspartate; NSAIDs, nonsteroidal antiin-flammatory drugs.
Data from Pepper A,M, Mercuri J,MM, Behery O,MM, et al. Total Hip and Knee Arthroplasty Peri-operative Pain Management. *0014030.* December 2018;6(12):e5 and Goode V, Morgan B, Muckler V, et al. Multimodal Pain Management for Major Joint Replacement Surgery. *National Association of Orthopaedic Nurses.* March/April 2019;38(2):150-156.

- Renal insufficiency
- Hepatic dysfunction
- Gastrointestinal dysfunction
- Hematological conditions
- Cognitive dysfunction

These comorbidities should be considered before the administration of any new medication.[10] In addition to oral medication, analgesic methods such as peripheral nerve blocks (PNBs) and local infiltration analgesia (LIA) can be used in combination to provide better pain relief.

Peripheral Nerve Blocks and Local Infiltration

Included in the term PNB are femoral nerve blocks, sciatic nerve blocks, and saphenous nerve blocks, either as a single shot or a continuous catheter. Compared with systemic methods alone, PNBs have proved to be effective in reducing pain, confusion, itching, and hospital length of stay.[27] LIA has shown significant pain relief and reduced opioid consumption compared with placebo.[13] However, the quality of evidence is low in LIA, because it is a newer technique; there is a need for higher-quality studies to determine its effectiveness.[28] Throughout the literature review for this article, there were many studies conducted using PNB and LIA; however, they are varied in their comparisons and outcomes, so a best practice cannot be identified at this time. A potential method for determining the best practice for a patient population and program would be to consider the advantages and disadvantages of each method (**Table 4**).

SOLUTIONS TO ADEQUATE PAIN CONTROL, NONPHARMACOLOGIC

Innovations in alternative therapies are gaining momentum in health care facilities nationwide. Hospitals are creating so-called comfort menus that provide options for pain management that do not include medications. The following examples are some of the alternative therapies that patients are encouraged to consider:

- Cryotherapy
- Transcutaneous electrical nerve stimulation
- Acupuncture
- Massage therapy
- Pet therapy
- Music therapy
- Visualization
- Aroma therapy
- Prayer/spiritual therapy
- Progressive relaxation
- Care channels
- Meditation
- Art therapy

In 2017, a meta-analysis of 5509 studies of nonpharmacologic interventions and their effectiveness was conducted, primarily focusing on continuous passive motion (CPM), preoperative exercise, cryotherapy, electrotherapy, and acupuncture.[5] The results of this meta-analysis in relation to pain relief and opioid consumption (**Table 5**) showed that electrotherapy and acupuncture showed moderate evidence of effectiveness. When specifically considering opioid consumption, electrotherapy reduced the amount of opioids consumed and acupuncture delayed the administration of opioids but not total amount consumed.[5]

Table 4		
Analgesic methods and their advantages/disadvantage		
Analgesic Method	**Advantages**	**Disadvantages**
PNB	Effective pain control. Moderate evidence in reducing opioid consumption. Standardized practice for medications used and placement technique	Motor impairment. Does not cover entire surgical site. Delay in surgical throughput for additional procedure
LIA	Effective pain control. Minimal systemic effects. No motor impairment. Early mobilization	Potential for increased surgical time. Effectiveness dependent on provider infiltration technique. No standardized cocktail for efficacy

PNB includes femoral nerve block and saphenous nerve block both single administration and continuous.
Data from Marques E, Jones H, Elvers K, et al. Local Anaesthetic Infiltration for Peri-Operative Pain Control in Total Hip and Knee Replacement: Systematic Review and Meta-Analysis of Short- and Long-Term Effectiveness. BMC Musculoskeletal Disorders. 2014;15(220):1471-2474; and Berninger M, Friederichs J, Augat P, et al. Effect of Local Infiltration Analgesia, Peripheral Nerve Blocks, General and Spinal Anesthesia on Early Function Recovery and Pain Control in Total Knee Arthroplasty. BMC Musculoskeletal Disorders. 2018;232(19).

Table 5 Nonpharmacologic meta-analysis results		
	Pain Relief	**Opioid Consumption**
CPM	Low to very low	Very low
Preoperative exercise	Low	Very low
Cryotherapy	Very low	Very low
Electrotherapy	Moderate	Moderate (reduce)
Acupuncture	Low	Moderate (delay)

Quality of the body of evidence.
Data from Tedesco D,M, Gori D,M, Desai K,P, et al. Drug-Free Interventions to Reduce Pain or Opiod Consumption After Total Knee Arthroplasty: A Systemic Review and Meta-analysis. 7501160. October 2017;152(10).

Cryotherapy

Cryotherapy is defined as the cooling of the skin at the surgical site or injury with either a bag of ice or an ice unit with cooling sleeve[5,29,30]; this is a common treatment of many painful conditions and is often used after TJR surgery. There are variations to cryotherapy, such as intermittent use versus continuous use and ice bag versus cooling sleeve. Which is the best method?

In randomized controlled trials with continuous use of the cooling sleeve, the most benefit was on postoperative day 2, with a reduction in pain, blood loss, and improved range of motion.[29,30] In a randomized trial with crossover, 2 groups were both administered oral narcotics at 2 time frames. At the first administration only, group 1 was given an intermittent cryotherapy treatment. At the second administration only, group 2 was given a cryotherapy treatment. The results showed no difference between the 2 groups' pain scores. Although they found no difference between the groups, the second group, which did not receive the initial treatment of cryotherapy, had higher pain scores before the second administration than the first treatment group.[29]

Although these studies show some benefit, the Cochrane Review states that[30]:

- There is reported decrease in pain on postoperative day 2, but there is no significant difference on days 1 and 3
- There is no evidence that shows a reduction in blood transfusion rates with the use of cryotherapy
- There is a potential in improved range of motion with cryotherapy
- There is very low evidence justifying the expense and inconvenience of an ice unit

Even though the literature does not support the use of cryotherapy as a standard of care, an important consideration is the patients' experience and their perception of the care they are receiving. There is a perceived value when they receive the unit to bring home, especially if they or family and friends have received one in the past.

Electrotherapy

Electrotherapy in orthopedics is typically delivered transcutaneously using conduction pads causing nerve stimulation. This therapy has been shown to reduce acute postoperative pain and opioid consumption and improve the long-term trajectory of pain.[5] In a randomized controlled trial, Adravanti and colleagues[31] found lower VAS scores in treated patients compared with the control group at months 1, 2, and 6 (**Table 6**). In a similar study, Moretti and colleagues[2] had similar findings. During Adravanti and colleagues'[31] study, the pain score in month 1 of the treatment group was the same as the control group at month 6.

Table 6
Electrotherapy visual analog scale score significance

	Adravanti et al[31] Study		Moretti et al[2] Study	
	P Value	Change (%)	P Value	Change (%)
Month 1	<.01	−61	<.0001	−63
Month 2	<.001	—	<.0001	—
Month 6	<.05	−90	<.001	−77

Follow-up versus baseline.

Data from Moretti B, Notarnicola A, Moretti L, et al. I-ONE Therapy in Patients Undergoing Total Knee Arthroplasty: A Prospective, Randomzed, and Controlled Study. BMC Musculoskeletal Disorders. 2012:13:88.

In addition to decreasing postoperative pain, there is a potential to improve postoperative swelling. There were statistically significant results (P<.01) in swelling reduction compared with baseline.[31] However, similar results were found in the control group, and there is minimal difference in swelling between the 2 groups at follow-up visits.[2,31] Considering these findings, electrotherapy seems to be an effective tool in reducing postoperative pain. Considerations in implementing this form of treatment into a TJR program are the cost of the unit, staff and patient educational needs, and compliance.

Acupuncture

There are limited studies on acupuncture and the TJR population. In one study, the subjects were in a fast-track program in which acupuncture was offered at the end of the physical therapy treatment. Short-term pain was reduced in 45% of the population and the moderate to severe pain was reduced from 41% to 15% after the acupuncture treatment.[9] The use of acupuncture did not reduce the amount of narcotics consumed but it did delay the time of the next administration.[5,9] In addition, it was effective in the acute phase but showed no long-term benefit for long-term pain outcome or trajectory.[5]

There are many considerations for introducing acupuncture into a TJR program:

- Cost
- Level of participation
- Physician and facility buy-in
- Available space for treatment
- Availability of a practitioner
- Facility and legal compliance
- Policies and procedures

Distraction therapies

Distraction therapy has been understudied in the orthopedic population. Examples of distraction therapy are pet therapy, music therapy, and art therapy. Despite minimal direct studies with this population, multiple studies regarding distraction therapies show a positive effect in patients with anxiety and depression.[32–35] Anxiety and depression are very common in patients undergoing TJR surgery.[15,32]

Pet Therapy

In the health care setting, pet therapy typically refers to dogs and their handlers. Dogs are the primary species used because of their accessibility. Although there are other species, such as cats, horses, reptiles, and birds, that can be therapy animals, they do not lend themselves as easily to an inpatient setting. Therapy dogs have been established as effective in treatment of patients with many different needs.[36]

A randomized controlled trial performed by Harper and colleagues[36] concluded that patients who received pet therapy had lower VAS scores (P<.001) after the third session. In addition to improved VAS scores, patients who participated in pet therapy gave an overall hospital rating significantly higher than the control group (P<.001).[36] There have been several studies that have shown the effectiveness of pet therapy in reducing depression and anxiety in patients.[36] There are many considerations in introducing pet therapy into a TJR program:

- Availability of trained animals and handlers
- Standard operating procedures of the organization
- Education around infection prevention

Music Therapy

Music therapy is an economical and viable option that is easily accessed in the clinical setting and has been shown to reduce anxiety in surgical patients.[32] Music therapy can be care channels, singing, and live music with the presence of a trained music therapist. There are limited studies that address the TJR patient population and music therapy. In a meta-analysis performed by Cochrane, music therapy was effective in providing short-term benefits to individuals with depression compared with usual treatment alone.[34] The review also found that music therapy influenced decreasing anxiety levels and improved function of depressed patients.[34]

Art Therapy

Art therapy can be defined as painting, drawing, coloring, modeling, and so forth and is another area that is understudied. A systematic review was performed searching for randomized and nonrandomized controlled trials using art therapy for the treatment of anxiety in adults. Abbing and colleagues[33] found that only 3 studies out of 776 publications met inclusion criteria for the review. The 3 trials that met criteria were determined to have a high risk of bias; at this time, no conclusions can be drawn about whether art therapy has an effect on anxiety. In a study performed by Doll and colleagues,[35] the effect of art therapy on mood, anxiety, and pain levels was evaluated in patients with cancer undergoing chemotherapy treatment; there were benefits observed immediately after the session and up to 72 hours thereafter.

Although art therapy needs further high-quality studies to confirm its effectiveness in reducing pain and anxiety, it continues to be a source of satisfaction for patients. In programs in which adult coloring has been trialed, the subjective evidence suggests that it can be a distraction during periods of pain at rest.

SUMMARY

TJR continues to be one of the most commonly performed and painful surgeries, causing moderate to severe pain in the acute postoperative period.[5,8–10] The difference between the experience of unrelieved pain and effective pain management continues to challenge health care providers. Managing the pain experience leads to improved outcomes.[3,10,12,13] The first step to managing the pain experience is identifying and managing modifiable risk factors for an improved pain experience. Managing the pain experience has many challenges, such as subjective pain assessment tools, side effects of medications, and fear of addiction. An environment had been created in which pain was the fifth vital sign, and opioids were the first-line treatment for decades. In the current paradigm of the opioid epidemic, government and state regulations are trying to rectify the effects of the old way of practice.

Patient education, multimodal therapies, and alternative therapies have been identified as critical first steps in decreasing the use of opioids in orthopedic surgery.[19] Focus has shifted to creating a reasonable pain expectation through mandatory preoperative patient and caregiver education. Preoperative education has also reduced the incidence of falls, complications, and hospital length of stay.[22–26] Extensive education of frontline nurses on alternative therapies such as multimodal medications, blocks, and distraction therapies is imperative for their ability to support their patients. The use of opioids over the course of decades cannot be overlooked when it comes to considering the practice changes for frontline nurses. Nurses are capable and well positioned to be active participants in creating solutions to the epidemic in their practices if appropriate time and resources are invested in their educational needs.

Multimodal analgesic medications, PNB, and LIA have become first-line treatments in the new paradigm. They have been effective in reducing narcotic use; however, there are many considerations to address. For multimodal medications, comorbidities, age, renal function, and hepatic function all need to be considered before administration. Also, there are no current guidelines or best practices in the selection of which medications to use, dosages, and frequency. Programs across the nation are learning from each other strategies for practice and adjusting to their own experiences with their patient population. PNB and LIA are effective in reducing the pain experience compared with normal treatment alone. However, current studies have either shown conflicting information or have fallen short of comparing the different nerve blocks with each other or LIA to find a best practice. Similar to multimodal approaches, practitioners learn from their colleagues and find what works for each facility and patient population. This area is one in which nursing can assist physicians in finding a best practice through research, collaboration, and reporting patient outcome measures.

Innovations in alternative therapies are gaining momentum in health care facilities nationwide. Hospitals are turning to comfort menus, creating an environment in which patients can choose alternative therapies that meet their specific cultural and personal needs. Comfort menus include alternative therapies such as prayer, meditation, music therapy, pet therapy, cryotherapy, acupuncture, visualization, art therapy, and massage therapy. In some facilities, these alternatives are listed on the comfort menu in lieu of a faces pain scale and last dose of pain medication administered. Instead of asking "What is your pain?" the question changes to, "How can we keep you comfortable?." These alternative therapies are understudied and are emerging as viable complimentary therapies to pharmacologic interventions alone. This approach also creates opportunity for nursing research and partnership with interdisciplinary teams to improve the pain experience.

Management of the patient's pain experience in orthopedics has come a long way in a short period of time. Advancements in technology, changes in medication management, adoption of adjunctive analgesics such as PNB and LIA, regulatory changes, and health care climate have all influenced this shift. There continues to be a gap between the pain experience and effective pain management and a gap in nursing practice from the old paradigm to the new paradigm. Closing these gaps requires an understanding of current and available therapies, potential alternative therapies, and a willingness to change.

DISCLOSURE

The authors have nothing to disclose.

REFERENCES

1. Lindberg MF, Miaskowski C, Rustøen T, et al. The impact of demographic, clinical, symptom, and psychological characteristics on the trajectories of acute postoperative pain after total knee arthroplasty. Pain Med 2017;18:124–39.
2. Moretti B, Notarnicola A, Moretti L, et al. I-ONE therapy in patients undergoing total knee arthroplasty: a prospective, randomized, and controlled study. BMC Musculoskelet Disord 2012;13:88.
3. Marques E, Jones H, Elvers K, et al. Local anaesthetic infiltration for perioperative pain control in total hip and knee replacement: systematic review and meta-analysis of short-and long-term effectiveness. BMC Musculoskelet Disord 2014;15(220):1471–2474.
4. Samuels J, Woodward R. Opportunities to improve pain management outcomes in total knee replacements. Orthop Nurs 2015;34:4–9.
5. Tedesco D, Gori D, Desai KR, et al. Drug-free interventions to reduce pain or opioid consumption after total knee arthroplasty: a systematic review and meta-analysis. JAMA Surg 2017;152(10):e172872.
6. Sloan M, Premkumar A, Sheth NP. Projected volume of primary total joint arthroplasty in the U.S., 2014-2030. J Bone Joint Surg Am 2018;100(17):1455–60.
7. Newswire P. Projected volume of primary and revision total joint replacement in the U.S. 2030 to 2060. Cision PR Newswire 2018. Available at: https://www.prnewswire.com/news-releases/projected-volume-of-primary-and-revision-totaljoint-replacement-in-the-us-2030-to-2060-300608386.html. Accessed May 20, 2019.
8. Gerbershagen HJ, Pogatzki-Zahn E, Aduckathil S, et al. Procedure-specific risk factor analysis for the development of severe postoperative pain. Anesthesiology 2014;120:1237–45.
9. Crespin DJ, Griffin KH, Johnson JR, et al. Acupuncture provides short-term pain relief for patients in a total joint replacement program. Pain Med 2015;16(6):1195–203.
10. Pepper AM, Mercuri JJ, Behery OA, et al. Total hip and knee arthroplasty perioperative pain management: what should be in the cocktail. JBJS Rev 2018;6(12):e5.
11. Schroeder D, Hoffman L, Fioravanti M, et al. Enhancing nurses' pain assessment to improve patient satisfaction. Orthop Nurs 2016;35:108–17.
12. Goode V, Morgan B, Muckler V, et al. Multimodal pain management for major joint replacement surgery. Orthop Nurs 2019;38(2):150–6.
13. Berninger MT, Friederichs J, Leidinger W, et al. Effect of local infiltration analgesia, peripheral nerve blocks, general and spinal anesthesia on early function recovery and pain control in total knee arthroplasty. BMC Musculoskelet Disord 2018;19:232.
14. Commonly Used Terms. Centers for Disease Control and Prevention. 2017. Available at: https://www.cdc.gov/drugoverdose/opioids/terms.html. Accessed May 20, 2019.
15. Greimel F, Dittrich G, Schwarz T, et al. Course of pain after total hip arthroplasty within a standardized pain management concept: a prospective study examining influence, correlation, and outcome of postoperative pain on 103 consecutive patients. Arch Orthop Trauma Surg 2018;138:1639–45.
16. Anderson I, Alger J. The tightrope walk, pain management and opioid stewardship. Orthop Nurs 2019;38(2):111–5.
17. Rosengren J. America's addiction to pain pills. AARP Bulletin 2017;9:10.

18. Sotomayor M. Senate passes sweeping legislation to combat opioid epidemic. NBC News 2018. Available at: https://www.nbcnews.com/politics/politics-news/senate-passes-sweeping-legislation-combat-opioid-epidemic-n908901. Accessed May 16, 2019.

19. Ariagno J, Combs B, Hughes M, et al. NAON Opioid Position Statement. National Association of Orthopaedic Nurses. 2019. Available at: http://www.orthonurse.org/p/do/sd/sid=4511. Accessed May 28, 2019.

20. Bodden J, Coppola C. Best practice guideline total hip replacement (arthroplasty). Chicago: SmithBucklin; 2018.

21. Mori C, Ribsam V. Best practice guideline total knee replacement (arthroplasty). Chicago: SmithBucklin; 2018.

22. Bergin C, Speroni K, Travis T, et al. Effect of preoperative incentive spirometry patient education on patient outcomes in the knee and hip joint replacement population. J Perianesth Nurs 2014;29(1):20–7.

23. Clarke HD, Timm VL, Goldberg BR, et al. Preoperative patient education reduces in hospital falls after total knee replacement. Clin Orthop Relat Res 2012;470(1): 244–9.

24. Huang SW, Chen PH, Chou YH. Effects of a preoperative simplified home rehabilitation education program on length of stay of total knee replacement patients. Orthop Traumatol Surg Res 2012;98(3):259–64.

25. Jones S, Alnaib M, Kokkinakis M, et al. Pre-operative patient education reduces length of stay after total knee replacement. Ann R Coll Surg Engl 2011; 93(1):71–5.

26. Yoon R, Nellans K, Geller J, et al. Patient education before hip or knee arthroplasty lowers length of stay. J Arthoplasty 2010;25(4):547–51.

27. Peripheral nerve blocks compared to other types of pain relief for people having total hip joint replacement surgery. Cochrane. 2017. Available at: https://www.cochrane.org/CD011608/ANAESTH_peripheral-nerve-blocks-compared-other-types-pain-relief-people-having-total-hip-joint-replacement. Accessed May 16, 2019.

28. Pain control using local anaesthetics to improve surgical results after shoulder, hip and knee replacement surgery. Cochrane. 2015. Available at: https://www.cochrane.org/CD010278/ANAESTH_pain-control-using-local-anaesthetics-improve-surgical-results-after-shoulder-hip-and-knee. Accessed May 16, 2019.

29. Witting-Wells D, Johnson I, Samms-McPherson J, et al. Does the use of a brief cryotherapy intervention with analgesic administration improve pain management after total knee arthroplasty? Orthop Nurs 2015;34(3):148–53.

30. Cold therapy following total knee replacement surgery. Cochrane. 2012. Available at: https://www.cochrane.org/CD007911/MUSKEL_cold-therapy-following-total-knee-replacement-surgery. Accessed May 3, 2019.

31. Adravanti P, Nicoletti S, Ampollini A, et al. Effect of pulsed electromagnetic field therapy in patients undergoing total knee arthroplasty: a randomised controlled trial. Int Orthop 2014;(38):397–403.

32. Giaquinto S, Cacciato S, Minasi E, et al. Effects of music-based therapy on distress following knee arthroplasty. Br J Nurs 2006;15(10):576–9.

33. Abbing A, Ponstein A, Hooren S, et al. The effectiveness of art therapy for anxiety in adults: a systematic review of randomised and non-randomised controlled trials. PLoS One 2018;13(12):e0208716.

34. Music therapy for depression. Cochrane. 2017. Available at: https://www.cochrane.org/CD004517/DEPRESSN_music-therapy-depression. Accessed May 28, 2019.

35. Doll M, Roshon S, Stone E, et al. Evaluation of art therapy on mood, anxiety, and pain levels in patients with cancer undergoing chemotherapy treatment. J Clin Oncol 2017;35(15).
36. Harper CM, Dong Y, Thornhill TS, et al. Can therapy dogs improve pain satisfaction after total joint arthroplasty? A randomized controlled trial. Clin Orthop Relat Res 2015;473(1):372–9.

Advances in Sports Medicine and Care of the Adolescent Athlete

Heather C. Barnes, DNP, APRN, CPNP, ONC*,
Angela C. Vanderpool, MSN, APRN, CPNP, ONC

KEYWORDS

- Sports medicine • Pediatric • Adolescent • Sports injuries

KEY POINTS

- The number of sports injuries in adolescents and children has greatly increased over the past 10 years to 15 years.
- The increases in youth sport participation and sports specialization has contributed to an increase in overuse and acute injuries.
- Nurses who care for adolescent and youth athletes have a unique opportunity to provide education as well as address key issues in this population.

HISTORIC REVIEW: EVOLUTION OF ATHLETICS FOR CHILDREN AND ADOLESCENT POPULATIONS

Over the past several decades there has been a dramatic change in the landscape of youth sports. Children and adolescents are less likely to be found participating in free play or neighborhood play and instead are involved in structured sport participation, led by a coach or adult leader.[1]

According to the 2008 National Council of Youth Sports report, an estimated 60 million youth ages 6 years to 18 years participate in organized sports.[2] Organized youth sports have evolved into a multi–billion-dollar industry.[3]

With the increase and widespread availability of organized youth sports there also has been a trend of single-sport specialization. By the time children have reached middle school and high school, they are less likely to participate in multiple sports[1,4]

FREQUENTLY SEEN CONDITIONS ASSOCIATED WITH YOUNG ATHLETES
Overuse Injuries

With the increase in youth sports participation, there naturally is an increase in injuries associated with participation. There are 2 types of injuries: acute injuries and overuse

Department of Orthopaedic Surgery and Musculoskeletal Science, Section of Sports Medicine, Children's Mercy Kansas City, 2401 Gillham Road, Kansas City, MO 64108, USA
* Corresponding author.
E-mail address: Hcbarnes@cmh.edu

Nurs Clin N Am 55 (2020) 239–250
https://doi.org/10.1016/j.cnur.2020.02.005
0029-6465/20/© 2020 Elsevier Inc. All rights reserved.

nursing.theclinics.com

injuries. Injuries resulting from overuse are estimated to be approximately 50% of all sport-related injuries and this may be underestimated in the literature.[5] Overuse injuries are defined as repetitive microtrauma to bone, muscle, or tendons without sufficient time to heal. Contributing factors to overuse injuries include sports specialization, overtraining, and a lack of participation in free play. Common overuse injuries in the lower extremity include Osgood-Schlatter disease, Sinding-Larsen–Johansson syndrome, Sever disease, and stress fractures. Common overuse injuries seen in the upper extremity include gymnast wrist, Little League elbow, and Little League shoulder.[6]

Several factors have been identified that may contribute to or increase the risk of sustaining an overuse injury. These factors often are described as intrinsic or extrinsic and some risk factors also can be described as modifiable and nonmodifiable. The American Medical Society for Sports Medicine identified intrinsic factors as those that are biological or psychosocial, such as growth-related factors, in contrast to extrinsic factors, which can be defined as external or environmental factors like training workloads and equipment that relate to the sport or activity.[5]

Nonmodifiable factors include age, gender, accelerated growth spurts, and history of previous injury. Previous injury has been identified as one of the strongest indicators for future injury.[5] Modifiable factors include flexibility, strength, and training volumes.

Osteochondritis dissecans (OCD) is considered an overuse injury that involves the subchondral bone with a risk of injury or disruption to the overlying articular cartilage.[7,8] Although the true etiology remains unknown, there are several factors that seem to be involved, including trauma, repetitive and overuse microtrauma, vascular insufficiency, and genetic predisposition.[8] The knee is the most common site where OCD lesions are found but they also can occur in the ankle, elbow, and shoulder.[9] If left untreated, there is an increased risk for development of osteoarthritis in the joint, which can cause lifelong physical limitations. Management of OCD lesions can result in a financial burden for patients and families from medical care costs as well as time lost from work.

Diagnosing OCD lesions is important to prevent long-term sequelae. Often patients with OCD lesions present with joint pain, stiffness, swelling, and locking.[8] Although OCD lesions can occur in adults, it most often is found in the skeletally immature population.[7] Male adolescents between 12 years to 19 years of age are affected most commonly, with frequency in children or adolescents who have played competitively for several years.[9] Clinical examination and radiographs of the knee, including anterior-posterior (AP), lateral, Merchant, and tunnel views, are most helpful in diagnosis (**Figs. 1–3**).[10] Once identified on radiographs, magnetic resonance imaging (MRI) may be obtained to determine if the lesion is stable or unstable, which is a predictor of how well the lesion will heal.[9,10]

Identifying the potential for healing of the OCD lesion is critical in developing a treatment plan. Lesion size, skeletal maturity, patient age, clinical symptoms, and signs of instability on the MRI are all important in the decision-making process.[9] Stable lesions in younger patients may be managed more conservatively by limiting activities for a period of time. Often stable lesions in children 12 years and older, as well as unstable lesions, may be evaluated further with an arthroscopy, the gold standard for identifying lesion stability.[9,10] At the time of the arthroscopy, drilling, internal fixation, or grafting of the lesion may be performed to stimulate healing of the lesion; this is critical in preserving the integrity of the articular cartilage.[10] Return to sports participation is dependent on recovery and can take anywhere from 3 months to 6 months or longer. Whether athletes are treated with conservative (nonoperative) or surgical management, they all have a period of activity restriction and require physical therapy for rehabilitation.

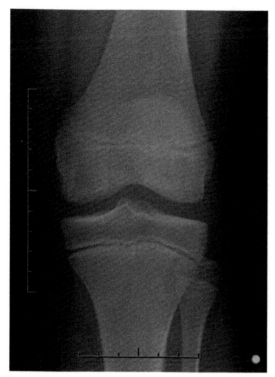

Fig. 1. OCD AP radiograph.

Once functional criteria have been met in therapy, they may begin the process of returning to play with recommendations by their therapist and treating physician.

Sports specialization has been identified as a contributing factor to an increased incidence of overuse injuries.[11–13] Sports specialization generally can be defined as participating in 1 sport to the point of exclusion of other sports. The American Orthopaedic Society for Sports Medicine (AOSSM) released a consensus statement in 2016 regarding early sports specialization recommendations and discussion around the potential detriment this trend may have on youth athletes.[11] AOSSM defined early sports specialization as participating in organized sports with intense training and/or competition for more than 8 months a year, participating in 1 sport to the point of exclusion of other sports, and involving prepubertal youth.[11] Sports specialization puts youth athletes at risk for injuries, burnout, physical and mental health concerns, and social isolation.[11–13]

Recommendations from the American Academy of Pediatrics Council on Sports Medicine and Fitness (2016)[11] include the following:

- Focus should be on fun.
- Participating in multiple sports until at least puberty may decrease chance of injury, burnout, and psychological stress.
- Specializing in a sport late adolescence may increase chance of achieving individual goals.
- Participating in multiple sports early and specializing later may promote lifetime sport participation and an emphasis on physical fitness.

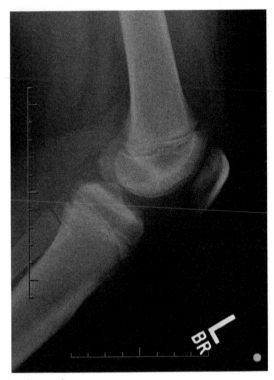

Fig. 2. OCD lateral radiograph.

- If early sport specialization occurs, ensure realistic goals and expectations of the athlete and the parents.
- Parents should be mindful and monitor participation to ensure best practices of coaching/training.
- Take a total of 3 months off a year from participation to focus on physical and psychological recovery.
- Athletes should have 1 day to 2 days off a week to decrease chance of injury.
- Intensive training should be closely monitored.

Sprains

Sprains account for a vast number of injuries related to sports participation in the adolescent population. Ankle sprains account for approximately 50% of all sport-related injuries.[14] Sprains occur as a result of stretching or tearing of a ligament between 2 bones. The most common age for ankle sprains to occur is during adolescence due to skeletal maturity. Younger athletes with open physis are at an increased risk to sustain a fracture through the physis because this area is considered a weak link. Sprains can be classified as lateral, medial, or high ankle sprains. Lateral ankle sprains are by far the most common.[14,15]

Sprains primarily occur as an acute injury or event. Lateral ankle sprains most commonly are associated with an inversion mechanism, medial ankle sprains with an eversion mechanism, and high ankle sprains occur with excessive rotational force.[14] A pop or snap often is heard or felt, with an immediate onset of swelling, bruising, pain, and difficulty bearing weight.

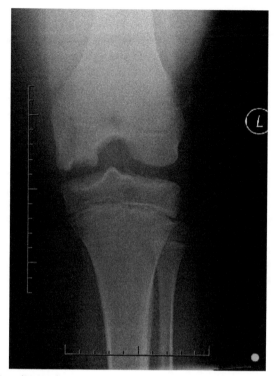

Fig. 3. OCD notch radiograph.

Careful physical examination should be performed to determine if radiographs are needed to evaluate for a fracture or more severe injury. Inspection of the skin for swelling, bruising, deformity, or concerns for skin integrity should be conducted. Active and passive range of motion should be evaluated as well as strength testing. Palpation of the bones, ligaments, and tendons is performed to identify areas of acute pain or tenderness.

Initial management of ankle sprains for an athlete should involve rest, ice, compression, and elevation (RICE). Lateral ankle sprain treatment may consist of a short period of immobilization and use of crutches if weight bearing is painful. Early range of motion and weight bearing can accelerate recovery.[14] Pain can be managed with acetaminophen and nonsteroidal anti-inflammatory drugs. Athletes should be referred to physical therapy to regain normal strength and range of motion and may return to play once they can achieve functional criteria for their sport. Length of time away from sport varies with severity of the sprain. Medial and high ankle sprains may require longer periods of immobilization and rehabilitation before an athlete is able to return to play.

Fractures

According to the most recent data from the National Collegiate Athletic Association, there are approximately 8 million students participating in high school sports.[16] The National Federation of State High School Associations reports a record number of participants in the 2017 to 2018 school year with an increase in participation having occurred for the previous 29 consecutive years.[17] With this increase in participation comes an increase in sport-related injuries. Sport-related fractures account for approximately 10% of all sport-related injuries in high school athletes.[18]

Sport-related fractures create a burden not only on the athlete but also the family. Athletes are sidelined from their activity, which can affect their mental well-being. They are subject to missed school days related to the injury, recovery, and rehabilitation. To diagnose fractures accurately, radiographic imaging is necessary and sometimes advanced imaging is required and can be costly. Swenson and colleagues[18] found that more than 17% of sport-related fractures required surgical intervention.

Growth plate fractures are unique to the pediatric and adolescent population because skeletal maturity occurs during the adolescent years. It is imperative that these types of fractures are diagnosed and managed accurately.

Ligamentous and Meniscal Injuries

Lower extremity injuries are common in youth and adolescent sports, making up approximately 40% of all injuries.[19] Anterior cruciate ligament (ACL) tears are only a fraction of those injuries but have been increasing steadily over the past 20 years at a rate of 2.3% annually. Pre-adolescent and adolescent female athletes are at the highest risk overall to sustain an ACL injury with the only exception in the 17 and 18 year-old males who exceeded females in rates of ACL tears. The highest incidence across both genders is in adolescents 16 years old to 18 years old.[20] These injuries can be life changing and result in months of rehabilitation, time off school and work, and inability to participate in sports. They also can be costly for a family and have long-term impact on an athlete's mental health and performance in school.[21]

The ACL is 1 of 4 ligaments that stabilize the knee by preventing the tibia from shifting forward in relation to the femur. It also helps prevent hyperextension, varus and valgus motion, and tibial rotation.[21] An intact ACL also protects the meniscus and articular cartilage when running, jumping, or stopping from shearing forces. An injury to the ACL increases the risk of injury to other structures in the knee, such as the meniscus, and increases the risk of osteoarthritis later in life.[22,23] A majority of ACL tears are a result of a noncontact injury during sports, often during cutting, pivoting, or landing after a jump.[23]

Diagnosing an ACL tear includes obtaining a good history. Often patients report feeling or hearing a pop, with the inability to continue playing. Most frequently they complain of pain, swelling from hemarthrosis, and often a feeling of instability.[21] Radiographs of the knee should be obtained to rule out a fracture, dislocation, or osteochondral injury in the young athlete with an acute knee injury. The clinic visit should include a thorough musculoskeletal examination, including specific orthopedic knee examination techniques, such as a Lachman test, pivot shift test, and anterior drawer test.[21] Pain, swelling, and anxiety can make it difficult to get a reliable examination. A good clinical examination can determine if the ACL is torn; however, if there are concerns with the examination, an MRI may be obtained to evaluate the ligaments further (**Figs. 4** and **5**).

Treatment of an ACL injury can be challenging to manage. It is not a surgical emergency but often there is a sense of urgency in the patient and family to return to pre-injury activities. Realistically, an ACL tear can be managed effectively either operatively or nonoperatively, if the family chooses. The goal is to provide a stable knee that functions well and allows leading a healthy, active lifestyle without further injury to the internal structures.[24] The decision for surgery is also dependent on the presence of other ligament injuries in the knee which may necessitate surgery to provide stability to the knee, including the posterior cruciate ligament, medial and lateral collateral ligaments, or the meniscus and articular cartilage in the knee. Age and demands placed on the knee by patients are additional factors to consider in the surgical decision process. Several graft types can be used, including hamstring,

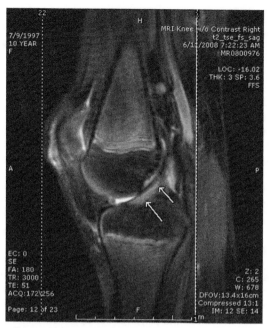

Fig. 4. Intact ACL radiograph. Arrows indicate the ACL.

quadricep, and bone patellar bone grafts. The type of procedure and graft also vary based on surgeon preference and skeletal maturity of the patient.[21] Whether a surgical or nonsurgical option is determined, high-quality rehabilitation is important in the recovery process, often taking 6 months to 12 months to return to sport participation.[24]

Meniscus Injuries

The frequency of meniscus injuries has increased steadily with the increased participation in sports. It is estimated that 80% to 90% of meniscus tears are related to sports participation in adolescent athletes but lower in the younger age bracket.[25,26] Meniscus injuries in children 10 years old and under are rare and often associated

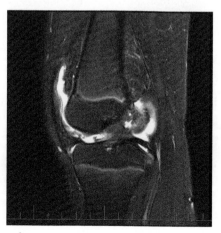

Fig. 5. Torn ACL radiograph.

with a discoid meniscus, a congenital anomaly. As adolescents increase in age, size, and speed, the competitive demands of the sport can result in more high-energy injuries.[26] Meniscus tears often are seen in combination with other knee injuries, including ACL tears, chondral injuries, and tibia fractures.[25] The largest group is seen in the adolescent population, with approximately 50% in conjunction with ACL tears.[27] This is concerning because the function of the meniscus is to load share and facilitate fluid motion and stability within the knee, similar to a shock absorber, protecting the articular cartilage and internal structures (**Fig. 6**).[26,28]

Diagnosis of a meniscus injury can be found on clinical examination and with a good history from the patient. Often there is a report of a twisting-type motion that resulted in knee pain, swelling, and giving way, sometimes with a report of a catching or locking sensation. On clinical examination, joint line tenderness and effusion often are seen. Clinical tests, such as the McMurray test and Apley test, also are effective diagnostic tools.[26] To rule out differential diagnosis, such as tendonitis, OCD lesion, patellofemoral instability, or tibial eminence fracture, knee radiographs are necessary. An MRI can be used to provide a definitive diagnosis and help rule out a loose body or other intra-articular injuries.

Treatment of a meniscus injury has changed over the years as knowledge of the function of the meniscus has developed and improved. Current research recommends treatment based on the location and type of tear. Many small, nondisplaced tears that are in the vascular portion of the meniscus may heal on their own with a period of rest from twisting, pivoting activities, and physical therapy. Tears that are large, are displaced, or cause persistent symptoms need an arthroscopy with débridement or repair of the tear.[26]

CRITICAL PROTOCOLS

There are few protocols or clinical practice guidelines published to assist health care providers in their decision making for management of sport-related injuries. The American Academy of Orthopaedic Surgeons (AAOS) published the "Management of

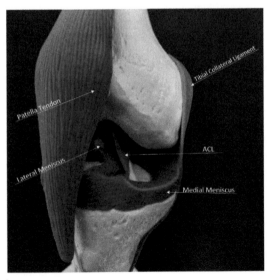

Fig. 6. Knee model.

Anterior Cruciate Ligament Injuries: Evidence-Based Clinical Practice Guideline" in 2014, which documented little evidence exists related to the skeletally immature patient; however, the recommendation supports surgical management versus nonoperative management to reduce future disability, instability, and injuries.[29]

In 2010, AAOS published a guideline and evidence support for the diagnosis and treatment of OCD. Reliable evidence did not exist to support recommendations; however, the opinion of the work group suggested symptomatic skeletally mature and immature patients with unstable or displaced OCD lesions be offered surgery. No specific recommendations could be made regarding methods for nonoperative treatment.[30] This lack of evidence highlights the need for further research to be conducted in the management of pediatric conditions.

SCREENING EXAMINATIONS
Preparticipation Examinations

Preparticipation examinations (PPEs) are recommended by a multitude of organizations prior to athletes' participation in a desired sport; however, there is no nationwide requirement regarding PPE completion in the United States.[31] Requirements for utilization of PPEs are left up to state high school associations to determine how they are implemented. The American Academy of Pediatrics along with the American Academy of Family Physicians, American College of Sports Medicine, American Medical Society for Sports Medicine, AOSSM, and the American Osteopathic Academy of Sports Medicine published a consensus document with recommendations on everything from when and where an examination should be conducted and who should conduct the examination to questions about medical and family history to a systems-based examination. There continues to be much debate regarding more advanced cardiac screening and the use of electrocardiograms as part of the PPE.[32–34] PPEs are not intended to exclude athletes from participation but rather to identify any risk factors for injury and remediate those factors when possible to allow for safe participation.

Suicide Screening

Suicide rates among adolescents are rising at an alarming rate. According to the Centers for Disease Control and Prevention, suicide is now the second leading cause of death among 10 year olds to 24 year olds.[35] An estimated 80% of individuals who died by suicide visited a health care setting within the year preceding their death.[36] This creates an important opportunity to implement quick screening of suicide risk within the health care community. Assessing the risk of suicide is crucial in identifying those at risk and is recommended by The Joint Commission.[37] The implementation of a screening process is one that should be thoughtful and connect patients and families at risk with appropriate resources. Approximately 50% of parents reported being unaware of their adolescent's suicidal thoughts during screening.[38] Education is paramount not only for health care providers performing the screening but also for families to value the importance of mental health and provide opportunities for further conversations regarding their child's overall well-being.[39]

NURSING IMPLICATIONS IN THE CLINICAL AND COMMUNITY SETTING

Nurses who care for adolescent and youth athletes in the clinical or community setting are positioned to educate families on many challenges that face this population in addition to providing care for injuries. Although many principles of managing acute injuries, such as sprains, fractures, and overuse injuries, are similar, the education that can be offered is invaluable. Patients and their families need to be educated and empowered to seek out information regarding being an athlete, such as sports specialization and sequelae that potentially can result from it, including but not limited to overuse injuries, burnout, and mental health concerns. With the increase in youth participating in organized sports, family dynamics have shifted to revolve around that sport and team. Sport participation can become the main social outlet for youth and their families. When an athlete sustains an injury and is prevented from participating, social isolation can be created for not only the athlete but also the entire family unit. Nurses need to be cognizant of this phenomenon to identify and provide support for the whole family. Nurses should advocate for preparticipation evaluations and encourage families to seek these from their medical home versus mass participation screenings. These evaluations provide an opportunity for the provider to have access to a more complete medical record history, and the adolescent may be more comfortable discussing sensitive issues.[34]

DISCLOSURE

The authors have nothing to disclose.

REFERENCES

1. Brenner JS. Sports specialization and intensive training in young athletes. Pediatrics 2016;138(3). https://doi.org/10.1542/peds.2016-2148.
2. Smucny M, Parikh SN, Pandya NK. Consequences of single sport specialization in the pediatric and adolescent athlete. Orthop Clin North Am 2015;46(2):249–58.
3. Youth team, league, and tournament sports: market shares, strategies, and forecasts, worldwide, 2018 to 2024. Youth Sports Market Research Study by WinterGreen Research. Available at: http://www.wintergreenresearch.com/youth-sports. Accessed May 30, 2019.
4. Myer GD, Jayanthi N, Difiori JP, et al. Sports specialization, part ii: alternative solutions to early sport specialization in youth athletes. Sports Health 2015;8(1):65–73.
5. Difiori JP, Benjamin HJ, Brenner JS, et al. Overuse injuries and burnout in youth sports: a position statement from the American Medical Society for Sports Medicine. Br J Sports Med 2014;48(4):287–8.
6. Arnold A, Thigpen CA, Beattie PF, et al. Overuse physeal injuries in youth athletes. Sports Health 2017;9(2):139–47.
7. Jones MH, Williams AM. Osteochondritis dissecans of the knee. Bone Joint J 2016;98-B(6):723–9.
8. Yellin JL, Gans I, Carey JL, et al. The surgical management of osteochondritis dissecans of the knee in the skeletally immature. J Pediatr Orthop 2017;37(7):491–9.
9. Cruz AI, Richmond CG, Tompkins MA, et al. What's new in pediatric sports conditions of the knee? J Pediatr Orthop 2018;38(2). https://doi.org/10.1097/bpo.0000000000001107.
10. Chambers HG, Shea KG, Carey JL. AAOS clinical practice guideline: diagnosis and treatment of osteochondritis dissecans. Am Acad Orthop Surg 2011;19(5):307–9.
11. Laprade RF, Agel J, Baker J, et al. AOSSM early sport specialization consensus statement. Orthop J Sports Med 2016;4(4). 2325967116644424.
12. Bell DR, Post EG, Biese K, et al. Sport specialization and risk of overuse injuries: a systematic review with meta-analysis. Pediatrics 2018;142(3). https://doi.org/10.1542/peds.2018-0657.

13. Brenner JS. Overuse injuries, overtraining, and burnout in child and adolescent athletes. Pediatrics 2007;119(6):1242–5.

14. Halstead ME. Pediatric ankle sprains and their imitators. Pediatr Ann 2014; 43(12). https://doi.org/10.3928/00904481-20141124-08.

15. Shah S, Thomas AC, Noone JM, et al. Incidence and cost of ankle sprains in United States Emergency Departments. Sports Health 2016;8(6):547–52.

16. Smeyers@ncaa.org. Estimated probability of competing in college athletics. NCAA.org - The Official Site of the NCAA. 2019. Available at: http://www.ncaa.org/about/resources/research/estimated-probability-competing-college-athletics. Accessed May 30, 2019.

17. NFHS. Available at: https://www.nfhs.org/articles/high-school-sports-participation-increases-for-29th-consecutive-year/. Accessed May 30, 2019.

18. Swenson DM, Henke NM, Collins CL, et al. Epidemiology of United States high school sports-related fractures, 2008-09 to 2010-11. Am J Sports Med 2012; 40(9):2078–84.

19. Sheu Y, Chen L-H, Hedegaard H. Sport and recreation related injury episodes in the U.S. population. Med Sci Sports Exerc 2016;48:868.

20. Beck NA, Lawrence JT, Nordin JD, et al. ACL tears in school-aged children and adolescents: has there been an increased incidence over the last 20 years? Pediatrics 2016;137(Supplement 3). https://doi.org/10.1542/peds.137.supplement_3.554a.

21. Labella CR, Hennrikus W, Hewett TE. Anterior cruciate ligament injuries: diagnosis, treatment, and prevention. Pediatrics 2014;133(5). https://doi.org/10.1542/peds.2014-0623.

22. Nessler T, Denney L, Sampley J. ACL injury prevention: what does research tell us? Curr Rev Musculoskelet Med 2017;10(3):281–8.

23. Wojtys EM, Brower AM. Anterior cruciate ligament injuries in the prepubescent and adolescent athlete: clinical and research considerations. J Athl Train 2010; 45(5):509–12.

24. Ardern CL, Ekås G, Grindem H, et al. 2018 International Olympic Committee consensus statement on prevention, diagnosis and management of paediatric anterior cruciate ligament (ACL) injuries. J ISAKOS 2018;3(2):66–82.

25. Shieh A, Bastrom T, Roocroft J, et al. Meniscus tear patterns in relation to skeletal immaturity. Am J Sports Med 2013;41(12):2779–83.

26. Kocher MS, Klingele K, Rassman SO. Meniscal disorders. Orthop Clin North Am 2003;34(3):329–40.

27. Werner BC, Yang S, Looney AM, et al. Trends in pediatric and adolescent anterior cruciate ligament injury and reconstruction. J Pediatr Orthop 2016;36(5):447–52.

28. Restrepo R, Weisberg MD, Pevsner R, et al. Discoid meniscus in the pediatric population. Magn Reson Imaging Clin N Am 2019;27(2):323–39.

29. Management of anterior cruciate ligament injuries evidence. Available at: https://www.aaos.org/globalassets/quality-and-practice-resources/anterior-cruciate-ligament-injuries/anterior-cruciate-ligament-injuries-clinical-practice-guideline-4-24-19.pdf. Accessed May 30, 2019.

30. Guideline on the diagnosis and treatment of osteochondritis dissecans. Available at: https://www.aaos.org/cc_files/aaosorg/research/guidelines/ocd_guideline.pdf. Accessed May 30, 2019.

31. Caswell SV, Cortes N, Chabolla M, et al. State-specific differences in school sports preparticipation physical evaluation policies. Pediatrics 2014;135(1): 26–32.

32. Harmon KG, Drezner JA, Oconnor FG, et al. Should electrocardiograms be part of the preparticipation physical examination? PM R 2016;8(3S). https://doi.org/10.1016/j.pmrj.2016.01.001.

33. Drezner JA, O'Connor FG, Harmon KG, et al. AMSSM position statement on cardiovascular preparticipation screening in atheletes: current evidence, knowledge gaps, recommendations and future recommendations. Br J Sports Med 2017;51: 153–67.

34. Mirabelli MH, Devine MJ, Singh J, et al. The preparticipation sports evaluation. Am Fam Physician 2015;92:371–376D.

35. Centers for Disease Control and Prevention, National Center for Injury Prevention and Control. Health, United States, 2016: with chartbook on long-term trends in health. 2015. Available at: https://www.cdc.gov/nchs/data/hus/hus16.pdf#019. Accessed February 20, 2018.

36. Ahmedani BK, Simon GE, Stewart C, et al. Health care contacts in the year before suicide death. J Gen Intern Med 2014;29(6):870–7.

37. A complimentary publication of The Joint Commission 6. Available at: https://www.jointcommission.org/assets/1/18/SEA_56_Suicide.pdf. Accessed May 30, 2019.

38. Jones JD, Boyd RC, Calkins ME, et al. Parent-adolescent agreement about adolescents' suicidal thoughts. Pediatrics 2019;143(2). https://doi.org/10.1542/peds.2018-1771.

39. Inman DD, Matthews J, Butcher L, et al. Identifying the risk of suicide among adolescents admitted to a children's hospital using the ask suicide-screening questions. J Child Adolesc Psychiatr Nurs 2019;32:68–72.

The Ever-Changing World of Limb Salvage Surgery for Malignant Bone Tumors

Kimberly K. Haynes, RN, DNP, MS, ACNS-BC, ONC, APRN*,
Howard G. Rosenthal, MD

KEYWORDS

- Bone sarcomas • Osteosarcoma • Ewing sarcoma • Chondrosarcoma
- Limb salvage surgery • Limb-sparing surgery

KEY POINTS

- Primary cancers of bone account for less than 0.2% of all cancers.
- Owing to the rarity of sarcomas, patients are treated by a multidisciplinary team of physicians and allied health professionals trained in treating sarcomas.
- Bone sarcomas are treated with surgery, sometimes chemotherapy and sometimes radiation therapy.
- Given the complexity of the treatment of sarcomas and the rarity of this diagnosis, patients are encouraged to be evaluated and treated in high-volume sarcoma centers by a multidisciplinary team.
- Bone sarcomas affect children and adults, accounting for 2% of all pediatric cancers and 1% of adult cancers.

INTRODUCTION

Sarcomas are cancers of the musculoskeletal system and form from connective tissue of the body such as bone, muscle, cartilage, nerves, blood vessels, and fat (mesenchyme or mesoderm); this is in contrast with carcinomas, which are derived from endodermal or ectodermal tissues. Sarcomas, both soft tissue and bone, are most prevalent in the extremities, but can occur anywhere. The American Cancer Society key statistics report states approximately 3500 new cases of bone sarcomas would be diagnosed in 2019 and 1660 patients would die from the disease.[1] The most common primary bone tumor in adults is chondrosarcoma and in children and young adults (<20 years) is osteosarcoma.[1] The most common overall bone tumor is osteosarcoma.

The University of Kansas Hospital Sarcoma Center, 10730 Nall Avenue, Suite 201, Overland Park, KS 66211, USA
* Corresponding author.
E-mail address: khaynes@kumc.edu

Rosenberg states, "Sarcomas of bone develop in all age groups. In many instances, however, there is a relationship between the patient's age and the specific location and type of tumor."[2] Osteosarcoma occurs in the second decade of life, whereas Ewing's sarcoma occurs most frequently in teens, but it can also be seen in younger children and in adults in their 20s and 30s.[3] Ewing tumors are most common in Caucasians and rarely occur in African Americans or other racial groups.[3]

The past 20 years have seen a remarkable shift in the outcomes of patients treated for sarcoma, both in the medical and surgical management of the disease, with more than 95% of patients now being treated in a limb savage manner and survival rates improving dramatically.

Primary bone cancers account for less than 0.2% of all cancers.[1] Owing to the rarity of sarcomas, it is best to have a patient with a sarcoma or a suspected sarcoma treated at a sarcoma center by physicians and allied health care professionals who specialize in sarcoma care. According to Henshaw, "It is widely accepted that a multidisciplinary approach is necessary to ensure the optimal care of patients with cancer, a complex disease that frequently requires a combination of treatments (eg, surgery, chemotherapy, radiation therapy) to offer patients a chance at long-term survival."[4] This team approach includes orthopedic and surgical oncologists, radiation oncologists, medical and pediatric oncologists, pathologists, and radiologists. Research has been done regarding increased survival rates for patients who are treated at sarcoma centers that treat a high volume of patients. Abarca and colleagues[5] found that centers that treat at least 10 sarcomas per year are considered high-volume centers and that these centers provided superior outcomes such with respect to fewer positive margins and long-term survival.

The multidisciplinary team is led by a musculoskeletal oncologist who is an orthopedic surgeon, fellowship trained in bone and soft tissue tumors, both benign and malignant. Other integral members of the team will include advanced practice nurses (APRN), registered nurses, nurse navigators, physical and occupational therapists as well as psychiatrists, physiologists, social workers, nurse case managers, and financial counselors. An accurate diagnosis requires the multidisciplinary team working together to correlate clinical information, radiographic features, histologic information, and treatment effects such as tumor necrosis, if the patient has undergone chemotherapy.[1] The multidisciplinary team works together to diagnose, formulate a treatment plan, and stage the tumor. Open communication between members of the treatment team allows for a personalized care for each individual patient in reference to their specific tumor type, anatomy, and personal needs. This process affords an improvement in overall outcome both from the oncological aspect as well as performance status.

DIAGNOSTIC WORKUP AND STAGING STUDIES

Diagnostic radiologic testing or staging studies ordered follow the National Comprehensive Cancer Network guidelines for the type of bone sarcoma diagnosed and are tailored to each patient. When a malignant bone tumor is suspected or known, certain radiologic testing can help with the diagnosis before a surgical biopsy or before further treatment, if the surgical biopsy is complete and diagnosis confirmed. A radiologic workup, also known as staging studies, includes a plain radiograph of the affected extremity and a MRI or computed tomography (CT) scan of the tumor with and without contrast. The plain film shows the current architecture of the bone and the MRI scan shows if there is a soft tissue component to the tumor and serves as the road map for further surgical planning (**Figs. 1** and **2**). A CT scan of the chest is

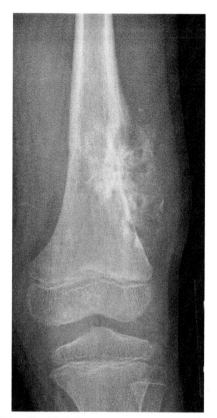

Fig. 1. Osteosarcoma of the distal left femur.

needed to look for spread of the tumor to the lungs (metastatic disease). If a sarcoma is going to spread, it will spread preferentially to the lungs. Sarcomas do not typically spread through the lymphatic system or spread to other locations in the body, except to the lungs; however, there are exceptions. Frequently, nuclear medicine imaging is conducted, such as a total body bone scan and PET scan. However, a PET scan is not considered standard of care for sarcoma care by insurance companies and therefore may not be a covered service by the patients' insurance company.

TREATMENT

Treatment modalities for bone sarcomas include surgery, chemotherapy, and radiation therapy. Depending on the diagnosis, staging studies and treatment protocol, chemotherapy and radiation therapy may or may not be used. The main treatment for bone sarcoma is surgery. Surgical procedures for bone sarcoma include amputation or limb salvage/limb-sparing surgery. The tumor must be removed in a wide en bloc fashion. This means removal of the tumor in 1 piece with a cuff of normal tissue surrounding and encompassing the entire tumor to ensure that every cell is indeed removed and that no tumor spillage occurs. This measure ensures that every sarcoma cell is removed with a clear margin. Any cancer cells that are left behind may grow and cause the tumor to recur.[6] Before the advances in chemotherapy and radiation therapy, and the technological advances in metal prosthetics used in limb salvage

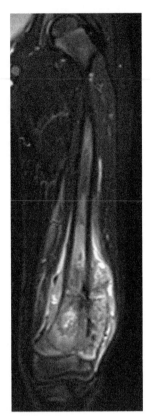

Fig. 2. MRI of an osteosarcoma left distal femur showing soft tissue involvement.

surgeries, amputation was the main surgical option to achieve a wide excision or complete removal of the tumor. Amputation of the limb is still used if the tumor cannot be removed without achieving clear margins with a limb salvage procedure. According to Cirstoiu and coworkers, the following are the essential requirements for limb-sparing surgery: "a subsequent tumor recurrence risk lower than after amputation; the possibility of achieving adequate resection margins; a durable reconstruction; low incidence of complications; and no negative effects on the adjuvant therapy protocol."[7]

Surgical Biopsy

If the patient has already had a biopsy at an outside institution, the pathology will be sent to the sarcoma center and may be examined by the sarcoma center pathologist. Because sarcomas are so rare, it is imperative that the diagnosis is accurate. Surgical biopsies may be an open biopsy, Tru cut needle biopsy, fine needle biopsy, or a CT- or ultrasound-guided needle biopsy. A Tru cut needle biopsy uses a needle with a large bore that will obtain a larger piece of tissue than a fine needle biopsy. An open biopsy and Tru cut needle biopsy produce a larger tissue sample, which is most beneficial. Given the rarity of the tumor type, a pathologist typically requires 1 cm^3 of tissue to perform all appropriate stains to ensure a correct diagnosis, grade, and analysis for molecular targeted therapies. Once the diagnosis is confirmed, the patient may be referred on to medical oncology and radiation oncology depending on the diagnosis.

Chemotherapy

Chemotherapy may be given before the definitive surgical procedure (neoadjuvant) or after the surgical resection (adjuvant). Neoadjuvant chemotherapy may be used if the tumor is high grade, if the patient has metastatic disease, if the tumor is close to or touching blood vessels or nerves, or if the tumor cannot be removed surgically. Chemotherapy for the treatment of osteosarcoma and Ewing's sarcoma has been shown to be effective in improving overall survival. Chemotherapy for chondrosarcoma has shown to not be effective and therefore is not in the treatment plan. Sarcoma patients with osteosarcoma or Ewing's sarcoma are treated by using a standardized protocol. Each patient may be assessed for entry into clinical trials available for certain patients with a sarcoma or based on a protocol specific to the institution or cancer type.

A protocol is a written procedure that has been confirmed by research to show benefits of increasing long term survival. Protocols for osteosarcoma and Ewing's sarcoma are different, and the chemotherapy drugs used are different. The chemotherapy drugs administered for osteosarcoma and Ewing's sarcoma need to be given at certain intervals and at certain doses depending on several factors including the patients' age, weight, and overall comorbidities. Also written into these protocols are time frames for repeating staging studies to assess treatment effect as well as time for the definitive surgical procedure. The protocols for osteosarcoma and Ewing's sarcoma include neoadjuvant treatment of 3 to 4 rounds to be completed before the definitive surgical procedure. After surgery, the patient waits to restart treatment (adjuvant chemotherapy) until the wound is healed. Because chemotherapy compromises the immune system, it is imperative that the patient's wound is healed before restarting chemotherapy, or complications of wound dehiscence and infection can occur. Because these patients will be undergoing bone surgery and have a metal implant such as a prosthesis or plate and screws, an infection in the surgical site could be catastrophic, leading to amputation. Adjuvant chemotherapy can last anywhere from 2 rounds to 6 or more rounds. The number of adjuvant rounds of chemotherapy depends on type of cancer, metastatic disease, tumor necrosis or amount of dead tumor in the surgical specimen, and the patient's overall tolerance.

Advances in chemotherapy are occurring daily and include immune checkpoint blockade therapy,[8] targeted therapy, and aspirin therapy as an adjuvant in osteosarcoma treatment.[9] Molecular targeted therapy is at the forefront of research currently and is partially defined as the ability to isolate a particular genetic protein or feature on the tumor cell and thus either repurpose a known drug or create a new drug to target this molecular aberration, which would result in ultimate demise of that cell.

Radiation Therapy

Radiation may or may not be used and can be delivered in several ways. Radiation is standard of care in Ewing's sarcoma but is not effective in osteosarcoma and chondrosarcoma. The most common form of radiation is external beam radiation. Other methods of radiation include stereotactic body radiation, brachytherapy, and intraoperative, and proton beam radiation.

External beam radiation can be given before surgical resection of the tumor (neoadjuvant) or after the tumor has been removed (adjuvant). Radiation therapy used before surgical resection will help to shrink the tumor away from critical structures and will form a rind around the tumor to help secure clear margins. This form of treatment occurs Monday through Friday for 5 weeks. Upon completion of the neoadjuvant radiation, the patient needs to wait several weeks to allow for the skin and soft tissues to heal and to allow for the cumulative effect of the radiation to occur. The radiation effects cause slowed wound healing and a greater chance of complications, such as wound dehiscence and wound infection. If external beam radiation is to be given after the definitive surgical resection, it starts approximately 2 weeks after surgery to allow for the surgical incision to heal. This form of radiation also occurs Monday through Friday and lasts up to 6 weeks. Just as with chemotherapy, radiation can cause wound complications such as blistering and peeling of the skin, wound breakdown (dehiscence), and/or delayed wound healing.

Brachytherapy is a form of delivery of radiation directly to the bed of the tumor where catheters are laid onto the wound bed during surgery and then filled with radiation seeds a few days later. This method allows radiation to be given directly to the wound bed and the dosage of radiation seeds inserted into each tube can be different if more radiation is needed in a certain part of the wound. This modality would be a more tailored radiation to a sarcoma bed, but would not necessarily ensure wider margins. After 3 to 4 days, the radiation seed sources are removed carefully and disposed of properly. The radiation catheters are removed easily in the patient's room or in the clinic.

Proton beam is a form of radiation that is becoming more popular, especially in pediatric patients. Proton beam technology allows for each radiation beam to be set to stop at a certain distance, such as at the edge or middle of the tumor, thereby sparing tissue surrounding the tumor. Ladr and Yock[10] state that "The physical properties of proton beam radiotherapy provide a distinct advantage over standard photo radiation by eliminating excess dose deposited beyond the target volume, thereby reducing both the dose of radiation delivered to nontarget structures as well as the total radiation dose deliver to a patient."[10] Proton beam therapy is very expensive and there are not many facilities currently that have this capability. However, if proton beam radiation helps to decrease long-term toxicities, especially in younger patients, such as second malignancies, the popularity will increase and hopefully the cost will decrease.[10]

Intraoperative radiation occurs in the operating room and is delivered directly to the wound bed once the tumor has been removed. This type of radiation is not as common owing to the cost of having an operating room equipped to provide the service.

ADVANCES IN THE TREATMENT OF SARCOMAS

The dawn of extremity bone sarcoma management was dominated by amputation as a standard of surgical treatment.[7] Advances in the surgical treatment of bone sarcomas over the last 50 years have occurred owing to advances in technology and research with respect to chemotherapy, radiation, surgical implants, and diagnostic imaging. Improvement in MRI scans, advent of PET scans, CT scanners with higher resolution and lower radiation emitted, and 3-dimensional imaging of tumors have all contributed to better surgical options.

Chemotherapy advances in the 1970s changed the survival rate in osteosarcoma from 17% to 60% to 70% or higher. The standard treatment for bone sarcomas in general includes neoadjuvant chemotherapy and sometimes neoadjuvant radiation, as well as surgical resection. Each treatment plan or protocol is tailored to that specific patient (**Table 1**).

LIMB SALVAGE SURGICAL OPTIONS

Surgical options have transitioned from amputation to limb salvage surgery, sometimes referred to as limb-sparing surgery, which is now the standard of care for the

Table 1
General treatment protocol, which may vary owing to grade and location of tumor

Bone Sarcoma	Surgery	Chemotherapy		Radiation	
		Neoadjuvant	Adjuvant	Neoadjuvant	Adjuvant
Osteosarcoma	Yes	Yes	Yes	No	No
Ewing's sarcoma	Yes	Yes	Yes	Yes	Yes
Chondrosarcoma	Yes	No	No	No	No

treatment of bone sarcomas. If any viable tumor is left behind, the sarcoma can grow and spread. The exceptions to limb salvage surgery would be if the tumor could not be completely removed without allowing for a functional extremity or if the tumor could not be removed with clear margins; in these cases, an amputation would be warranted.

Reconstruction of bone when a tumor has been removed can be achieved in several ways, depending on tumor location and the patient's age and overall health status. To eradicate the tumor with clear margins requires the resection of diseased bone or the joint involved in the tumor. Limb salvage surgical procedures to reconstruct the defect include the following: endoprosthesis, human bone transplant (vascularized fibula graft) using the patient's own bone (autograft), allograft (cadaver bone), alloprosthesis (metal prosthesis and allograft combined), noninvasive expandable prosthesis, and rotationplasty. Metal plates and screws can be used, as well as other adjuvant treatments such as cryosurgery, phenol, manmade bone grafts, human cadaver bone graft, and methyl methacrylate (bone cement). Carbon fiber plates, in contrast with stainless steel or titanium, are radiolucent on radiographs, allowing the surgeon to be able to see the surgical defect site through the plate, which helps with monitoring for local recurrence.

Endoprosthesis

Endoprosthetic reconstruction is a fairly new technology whereby the resected portion of bone, joint, and ligaments are reconstructed using an artificial implant that replicates the part removed. As little as 25 years ago, these implants required custom design, fabrication, and development. With technological advances, metal prostheses are now segmental and can be customized during the actual surgery to fit each patient individually, meaning that there is no wait time. The segments are available in many sizes and a custom fit to the patient can occur in minutes (**Fig. 3**). The prosthesis can also be a total bone replacement, such as a total femur replacement or a total humerus replacement. These implants can encompass more than 1 joint and the stem can be cemented in or cementless. The stems can be different shapes and sizes and can be coated with hydroxyapatite or hydroxyapatite tricalcium phosphate, which helps to stimulate bony ingrowth into the stem for added support. Cementless fixation is preferred, but if the bone quality is poor a cemented stem is used.[7] These prostheses are stronger and are lasting 20 years and sometimes longer. The life of the prosthesis also depends on how active the patient is and how much abuse the reconstructed limb receives. One of the greatest challenges with using an endoprosthesis is soft tissue attachments, such as tendons and ligaments. Attaching these soft tissue components to metal can be done with suturing, plate and screw fixation, or mesh. In addition, there is new potential on the horizon for promoting soft tissue ingrowth into the metal[7] (**Figs. 4–6**).

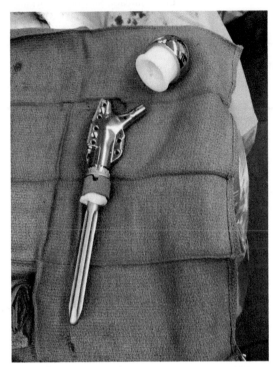

Fig. 3. Proximal right femur replacement.

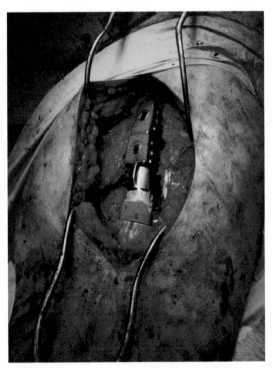

Fig. 4. Proximal right femur with the prosthesis implanted.

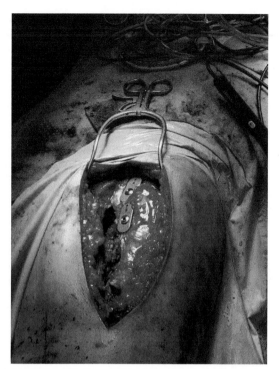

Fig. 5. Proximal right femur with the prosthesis implanted and soft tissue approximation.

Contraindications for use of the endoprosthesis may include young age and skeletal immaturity; tumor that encompasses the bone, blood vessels, and nerves; poor bone quality; inadequate soft tissue coverage; and even pathologic fracture through the tumor, which will have caused contamination of the soft tissues. Failures include mechanical failure, such as loosening of the prosthesis, and nonmechanical failure, such as infection or tumor progression.[7]

Vascularized Bone Grafts

Reconstruction of long bone defects can be challenging. For those tumors occurring in the diaphysis or shaft portion of the long bones, reconstruction may be carried out by

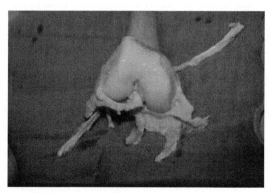

Fig. 6. Allograft with soft tissue attachments.

using a biological solution. Using the body's expendable bones such as the fibula, ribs, portion of ilium, and clavicle, one can harvest these expendable bones on the vascular pedicle and incorporate them into the long bone defect where a tumor was resected. The vascular pedicle to the bone graft can be reanastomosed to the host accompanying blood vessels, thereby achieving a vascularized bone graft or living bone transplantation. The vascularized bone graft tends to remodel and heal more promptly than an allograft and remodels over time to completely replace the resected segment of bone. The complication rate for vascularized bone graft is low and postoperative radiographic monitoring is easier because there are no large segments of metallic prostheses that cause artifact on various imaging modalities.

The surgical technique is more complicated and technically more difficult, and commonly requires a microvascular surgeon for the harvesting of the bone as well as the reanastomosis. These procedures should be carried out in centers with the appropriately trained personnel, such as microvascular surgeons who perform a high volume of microvascular surgery. Nonvascularized fibula grafts can be used; however, a comparison study performed by Estrella and Wang[11] found vascularized fibula grafts were 4 times more likely to unite compared with nonvascularized fibula grafts.[11] Advantages of the vascularized fibula graft include low morbidity at the donor site, durability, bone healing potential, immediate stability owing to its cortical stiffness, and its ability to hypertrophy to near the size of the host bone.[11,12] Complications that can occur include nonunion, fractures of fibula graft, hardware failure, infection, loss of vascular viability, and limb length discrepancy.[13,14] A disadvantage is the long period of restricted weight bearing.

Segmental Bone Transplant

This technique uses distraction osteogenesis. This procedure is used when the tumor occurs in the diaphysis or metaphysis of long bones or approaches the epiphysis. Stabilization of the bone occurs with use of an external fixator.[7] This procedure transports normal bone slowly at a calculated rate ranging from 0.5 to 2.0 mm/d,[15,16] to fill in the defect left when the cancerous bone is removed. Yang and colleagues[15] reported on 2 cases of successful bone transportation that occurred using distraction osteogenesis. These authors feel that this procedure has a shorter operation time, is a simpler procedure, and has fewer complication risks.[15] Yang and colleagues[15] state that "The use of bone transport distraction generally precludes the requirement for internal fixation and prosthesis implantation; therefore, this significantly minimizes the chances of wound infection."[15] The longer the external fixator was in place, the greater the chance of complications with infection and soft tissue constraints. Disadvantages include a higher risk of infections owing to immunosuppression from chemotherapy, muscle contraction, and nerve damage; delayed healing; and the time burden on the patient.[7] However, the benefits include restoration of limb length discrepancies, easier management of infection, and good functional outcomes owing to the use of host bone.[7]

Cadaver Bone Transplant (Allograft) and Alloprosthesis

Allograft reconstruction, or the transplantation of living cadaveric bone into the host, was a commonly used reconstruction option in the 1980s and 1990s. Once the surgical resection of the bone sarcoma was complete, the bony defect was reconstructed using a structural fresh frozen allograft, that being either intercalary or osteoarticular.[17] Aponte-Tinao and colleagues[17] state that, "If the epiphysis was removed with the tumor resection, the joint was reconstructed by attaching the ligaments to the corresponding allograft tissues to improve stability" (see Fig. 6). If a limb length discrepancy is expected, an extra 1 to 2 cm of length would be added to the allograft to allow for growth of the child.[17] This mode of reconstruction was a good option in that it reconstructed the joint, muscles, ligaments, and tendons; however, complication rates were high and over the years this mode of reconstruction has been mostly replaced with endoprostheses. After failure of the allograft, the use of the allograft and prostheses together became popular for a short time (**Fig. 7**). The allograft around the knee could be ordered with all soft tissue attachments, allowing for a more anatomic reconstruction. The metal prosthesis provided the structural support. However, as advancements in the metal prosthesis progressed, this type of reconstruction became less popular.

Noninvasive Expandable Prosthesis

The custom fit prostheses work well in adults, but the problem for many years occurred in skeletally immature children. The original development of the minimally invasive expanding prosthesis allowed small segmental adjustments to be added to the metal prosthetic implant over time as the child grew. The frequent surgeries to add the metal segments put the patient at risk for infection. Then came the development of noninvasive expanding prostheses, which are now used frequently. Built into the prosthesis is the ability for the prosthesis to extend to a certain length. The prosthesis is lengthened by the use of an externally applied magnetic field.[18] Gundavda and Agarwal state that "The noninvasive expandable prosthesis is an ideal implant for children undergoing limb salvage surgery for bone sarcoma who are expected to have more than 3 cm of limb length discrepancy at maturity."[18] As the patient grows, the prosthesis gets lengthened by a few millimeters every few months. The noninvasive lengthening procedure is accomplished in the office, without anesthesia, using a radio transmitter encircling the limb sending a current that powers a gear mechanism within the implanted prosthesis, thereby achieving lengthening. This procedure can lengthen a patient typically between 4 and 8 mm over a less than 30-minute period, enabling the patient to maintain equal limb lengths throughout growth and be continuously fully weightbearing. The benefit is minimal pain with no loss of function.[18]

Rotationplasty

Limb salvage or limb sparing is the standard of care for bone sarcomas, if the tumor can be removed in its entirety and with clear margins. In children less than 10 years of age, there is another option besides the noninvasive expandable prosthesis called a rotationplasty. A rotationplasty is a double-level amputation that removes the

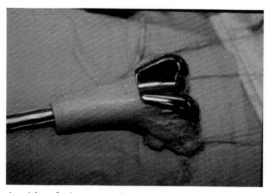

Fig. 7. Alloprosthesis with soft tissue attachments.

diseased portion of the child's bone around the knee joint. The knee joint (distal femur and proximal tibia and fibula) is removed except for the blood vessels and nerve. The lower section of the limb (tibia/fibula) is then rotated 180° and connected to the remaining femur with plates and screws and the ankle joint now becomes the knee joint (**Fig. 8**). The location of the new knee joint is calculated by the amount of growth the child has left. The child can function as a below knee amputee and as the nonsurgical leg of the child grows, the knee joint on the surgical leg begins to even out with the other knee joint. The goal when the child reaches skeletal maturity is to have the ankle joint be functioning well and be at the same height as the knee of the nonsurgical leg. Cirstoiu and colleagues[7] state that "The main reason a rotationplasty is sometimes preferred over a radical ablative procedure is that it ensures better functional results by providing a longer residual limb with better fitting for an external prosthesis."

Owing to the radical nature of this procedure, certain criteria need to be met before the procedure is performed. According to Potter,[19] there must be a functioning ipsilateral ankle and the sciatic nerve must be spared. He also states that a local prosthetist must be able to provide the specialized prosthesis and, most important, the patient and family should undergo extensive education and counseling.[19] It can be beneficial to have the patient and family meet another patient who has successfully undergone the procedure and is functioning well. This measure allows the patient and family to have an opportunity to get questions answered on a personal level. Although the procedure is disfiguring, patients generally do very well. The research study by Gradl and colleagues[20] looked at the long-term functional outcomes and quality-of-life scores. They found that patients who had undergone rotationplasty were enjoying a high quality of life and good functional outcomes.[20] Many patients can participate in a variety of sporting activities, limited by the prosthesis.[19,20]

COMPLICATIONS

Complications after surgery for a bone sarcoma can be catastrophic, including infection; nonunion of the allograft–host bone interface; periprosthetic, prosthetic, or allograft fracture; loosening of the metal hardware; limb length discrepancy; malalignment; and multiple revision surgeries. Owing to neoadjuvant chemotherapy and/or radiation, the patient is at added risk for infection and wound breakdown. Infection occurring around a metal prosthesis can be very difficult to eradicate and the patient may have to undergo several surgeries, including removal of the prosthesis or metal to maintain length while attempting to eradicate the infection. The patient needs

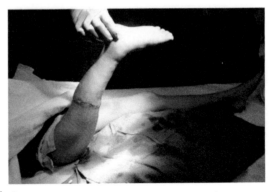

Fig. 8. Rotationplasty.

to be educated to the signs and symptoms of infection and be instructed to call the office immediately if any of the signs occur. If a wound infection occurs, depending on the severity, it may be able to be treated initially with antibiotics. If the infection does not clear, a surgical irrigation and debridement may necessary to wash out the wound bed and remove any necrotic or infected tissue. If the infection goes down to the bone, the prosthesis may need to be removed and replaced by a cement spacer impregnated with antibiotics for several months. If the infection clears, a new prosthesis can be reimplanted. If the infection does not clear, an amputation may be needed.

Another complication that can occur is loosening or failure of the metal prosthesis or plate and screws. If this happens, then the prosthesis or hardware will be removed and another surgical reconstruction will need to take place. The problems that can occur with repeated surgeries include, infection, bone loss, nerve damage and increased scar formation. As mentioned elsewhere in this article, an amputation may be necessary if reconstruction is not a viable option.

NURSING CARE OF THE PATIENT

Any patient with cancer will need help navigating the cancer world, a new world to the patient, full of unknowns. Patients with cancer are vulnerable, afraid, uneducated with respect to the diagnosis, and come from a variety of cultural and socioeconomic backgrounds.[21] A multidisciplinary team approach from a dedicated sarcoma center offers the patient with a sarcoma the best chance for long-term survival. As the patient is being treated by the physicians, the nurses are caring for the patient daily. Having nurses who understand the issues related to bone cancer surgery, chemotherapy, and radiation will lead to much better patient outcomes. This team should include, in addition to the sarcoma clinic nurses, nursing staff in the operating room and on the surgical floor. Continuity of care influences the patient experience in many positive ways. Having nurses who understand what the patient has been through and will have to go through after surgery is imperative.

A nurse navigator may be the first contact the patient has after learning of their cancer diagnosis or possible cancer diagnosis. The nurse navigator will help the patient to get timely care by assisting with the retrieval of medical records and films, getting appointments set up with other medical providers, and setting up appointments for financial counselors, as well as making referrals to a psychologist or psychiatrist if needed. Research on navigation has shown that "patient navigators can play a significant role in helping patients with cancer access care across an extremely complex continuum.[22]

The navigator assists with setting up the appointments for medical oncology and radiation oncology. A patient with sarcoma may not need both treatments, but can benefit by meeting with these physicians to get a better understanding of why a treatment is being recommended or not. The medical oncologist and radiation oncologist discusses the pros and cons of treatment as well as the potential for increasing survival rates. The navigator also assists in arranging for genetic testing, nutritional evaluation, and other adjuvant options available to the patient with a sarcoma. Additionally, the navigator acts as the liaison to all involved with the patient, including tumor board conferencing and social support.

An APRN can help to guide the patient's care. Three types of APRNs—clinical nurse specialists, nurse practitioners, and certified registered nurse anesthetists (CRNA)—partner with the surgical, medical, and radiation oncologists to help provide high-quality patient care. Clinical nurse specialists and nurse practitioners talk with the patient after the diagnosis to clarify what information the patient may not have understood. Patients are often overwhelmed at the onset of their treatment, and the APRN can help to manage the patient as the patient undergoes treatment. The APRN rounds on the patient in the hospital and sees the patient in the clinic. The clinic nurses consult with the APRN when difficult patient problems or concerns arise. Having the clinic nurses be knowledgeable is the mainstay of a good sarcoma clinic. The staff nurses caring for the patient in the hospital must be educated about the surgical procedure to ensure safe postoperative care along with maintaining any restrictions that are needed. The APRNs and registered nurses at the medical oncology and radiation oncology offices play an integral and collaborative roll with the APRN and registered nurses at the Orthopedic Oncology surgeon's office. All team members must work together to ensure that the patient gets the highest standard of care so the patient can achieve the best long-term outcome.

The CRNA cares for the patient during the surgical procedure. Rosenthal and Haynes[23] state that "the CRNA must understand how the use or certain bone grafts and bone fillers affect the patient."[23] Polymethyl methacrylate or bone cement can cause cement emboli and exothermic burns that can harm the patient. Also with the use of liquid nitrogen gas emboli and vascular injury can occur and the CRNA must be ready to act immediately if one of these events occurs.[23]

Registered nurses in the hospital need to be knowledgeable on the care of a patient with sarcoma. The specialized surgical procedures mentioned elsewhere in this article require expert and diligent nursing care. A patient undergoing surgery for a bone sarcoma will most likely be placed on an orthopedic unit in the hospital. Nurses on an orthopedic unit will have experience with caring for patients with total joint replacements, which is integral. Most bone sarcomas occur around a joint; therefore, a patient undergoing an endoprosthetic replacement has many of the same postoperative instructions as a patient undergoing total joint replacement. However, a patient with sarcoma undergoing an endoprosthetic replacement, rotationplasty, vascularized fibula graft, or internal fixation with plates and screws will have specific care instructions regarding range of motion, weightbearing status, and ambulation restrictions.

Other allied health professions, such as physical therapy, occupational therapy, and social work, all with experience in sarcoma care, play an integral part in providing expert care to a patient with sarcoma. Mental health professionals such as psychiatrists and psychologists are a part of the sarcoma team. Physiatrists and prosthetists are involved in the long-term rehabilitation of the pediatric patients who have undergone a rotationplasty or if a patient ended up with an amputation.

SUMMARY

Patients with a sarcoma have many options when undergoing treatment for a sarcoma of the extremity. Each option has pros and cons associated with the procedure. Upon meeting the patient, education begins regarding definitive surgical procedures that are possible. A detailed discussion with the patient regarding long-term goals regarding functional outcomes needs to take place weeks before the definitive surgical procedure is planned so the physician and patient can feel comfortable with the surgical plan.

For adults, endoprosthetic replacement is the standard of care as long as clear margins can be achieved. Allografts or alloprosthesis can be used, but more complications can occur with fracture of the allograft. The use of a vascularized fibula graft is an excellent biological option, but can have problems with nonunion, plus morbidity from the fibula graft donor site, albeit small. All tumors must be removed with a cuff of normal tissue surrounding the mass with the goal of maintaining a functional limb. If the tumor cannot be removed with clear margins, amputation will be recommended. A standard endoprosthesis cannot be used in skeletally immature patients owing to continued growth that will occur. Pediatric patients have options for rotationplasty and bone transportation by osteogenic distraction, as well as the noninvasive growing prosthesis. Each technique has unique benefits and disadvantages. A rotationplasty can offer excellent function, but can have psychological effects owing to the disfigurement that occurs from the procedure. The noninvasive growing prosthesis is also an excellent reconstructive option, but can have issues with hardware failure and nerve, skin, and muscle damage owing to the numerous lengthening that occur as the child grows. This option may also require another surgery to change out the growing prosthesis to a standard endoprosthesis as the patient reaches skeletal maturity.

Chemotherapy and radiation therapy can cause long-term issues that need to be monitored closely. Chemotherapy can cause infertility, cardiac issues, kidney problems, neuropathy, and second malignancies. Radiation therapy causes permanent skin changes and can cause nerve damage, and can also cause secondary malignancies. Offering a sarcoma support group and/or survivorship clinic can help patients to manage these potential side effects so they can live their best life possible.

DISCLOSURE

The authors have nothing to disclose.

REFERENCES

1. Key statistics for Ewing tumors. Available at: https://www.cancer.org/cancer/ewing-tumor/about/key-statistics.html. Accessed May 25, 2019.
2. Rosenberg AE. Bone sarcoma pathology: diagnostic approach for optimal therapy. Am Soc Clin Oncol Book 2017;37:794–8.
3. Key statistics for Ewing tumors. Accessed May 25, 2019.
4. Henshaw RM. In: Henshaw RM, editor. Sarcoma: a multidisciplinary approach to treatment. Cham (Switzerland): Springer International Publishing; 2017. p. 3–9.
5. Abarca T, Gao Y, Monga V, et al. Improved survival for extremity soft tissue sarcoma treated in high-volume facilities. J Surg Oncol 2018;117(7):1479–86.
6. Surgery for bone cancer. Available at: https://www.cancer.org/cancer/bone-cancer/treating/surgery.html. Accessed March 26, 2019.
7. Cirstoiu C, Cretu B, Serban B, et al. Current review of surgical management options for extremity bone sarcomas. Efort Open Rev 2019;4:174–82.
8. Thanindratarn P, Dean DC, Nelson SD, et al. Advances in immune checkpoint inhibitors for bone sarcoma therapy. J Bone Oncol 2019;15:100221.
9. Yang Y, Han L, He Z, et al. Advances in limb salvage treatment of osteosarcoma. J Bone Oncol 2018;10:36–40.
10. Ladra MM, Yock TI. Proton radiotherapy for pediatric sarcoma. Cancers 2014; 6(1):112–27.
11. Estrella EP, Wang EH. A comparison of vascularized free fibular flaps and nonvascularized fibular grafts for reconstruction of long bone defects after tumor resection. J Reconstr Microsurg 2017;33(3):194–205.
12. Miyamoto S, Fujiki M, Setsu N, et al. Simultaneous reconstruction of the bone and vessels for complex femoral defect. World J Surg Oncol 2016;14(1):291.
13. Ghoneimy AME, Sherbiny ME, Kamal N. Use of vascularized fibular free flap in the reconstruction of the femur in pediatric and adolescent bone sarcomas: complications and functional outcome. J Reconstr Microsurg 2019;35(2):156–62.

14. Manfrini M, Bindiganavile S, Say F, et al. Is there benefit to free over pedicled vascularized grafts in augmenting tibial intercalary allograft constructs? Clin Orthop Relat Res 2017;475(5):1322–37.
15. Yang Z, Jin L, Tao H, et al. Reconstruction of large tibial bone defects following osteosarcoma resection using bone transport distraction: a report of two cases. Oncol Lett 2016;12(2):1445–7.
16. Wang W, Yang J, Wang Y, et al. Bone transport using the Ilizarov method for osteosarcoma patients with tumor resection and neoadjuvant chemotherapy. J Bone Oncol 2019;16:100224.
17. Aponte-Tinao LA, Albergo JI, Ayerza MA, et al. What are the complications of allograft reconstructions for sarcoma resection in children younger than 10 years at long-term followup? Clin Orthop Relat Res 2018;476(3):548–55.
18. Gundavda MK, Agarwal MG. Growing without pain: the noninvasive expandable prosthesis is boon for children with bone cancer, as well as their surgeons! Indian J Orthop 2019;53(1):174–82.
19. Potter BK. CORR Insights(R): how much clinical and functional impairment do children treated with knee rotationplasty experience in adulthood? Clin Orthop Relat Res 2016;474(4):1005–7.
20. Gradl G, Postl LK, Lenze U, et al. Long-term functional outcome and quality of life following rotationplasty for treatment of malignant tumors. BMC Musculoskelet Disord 2015;16:262.
21. Case MA. Oncology nurse navigator. Clin J Oncol Nurs 2011;15(1):33–40.
22. Campbell C, Craig J, Eggert J, et al. Implementing and measuring the impact of patient navigation at a comprehensive community cancer center. Oncol Nurs Forum 2010;37(1):61–8.
23. Rosenthal H, Haynes K. In: Henshaw RM, editor. Sarcoma a multidisciplinary approach. Cham (Switzerland): Springer International Publishing; 2017. p. 335–50.

Excellence in Patient Education

Evidence-Based Education that "Sticks" and Improves Patient Outcomes

Carolyn Crane Cutilli, PhD, RN-BC[a,b,*]

KEYWORDS

- Patient education process • Health literacy • Patient teaching • Evidence-based
- Patient engagement • Patient-centered • Health literacy universal precautions
- Multimodal

KEY POINTS

- Patient education is a process with 4 components (assessment, planning, implementation, and evaluation). Each component must be equally addressed by the nurse for excellence in patient education.
- Patient education is an "art" and "science' using nuances and evidence-based strategies to effectively educate. Assessment and evaluation often require nuanced approaches (motivational interviewing, teach back) to engage patients/caregivers, whereas planning and implementation rely more on evidence-based strategies such as the Patient Education Materials Assessment Tool.
- Successful patient education incorporates Health Literacy Universal Precautions as well as knowledge from other fields such as marketing. Nurses should provide education that is simple, patient centered, and multi-modal to meet the health literacy needs of patients/caregivers.

INTRODUCTION

For nurses, patient education is a large part of standard care; teaching approaches have developed over time.[1] To support patient self-management and caregivers, it is essential that nurses provide health education in a manner that engages the patient/caregivers and is individualized.[2] Executing excellent patient education is an "art" and "science"—nuanced and evidence based. A knowledgeable and skilled nurse uses the patient education process that mirrors the nursing process: assessment, planning, implementation, and evaluation.[1] This process provides the foundation for any form of

[a] Hospital of the University of Pennsylvania, Philadelphia, PA, USA; [b] American International College, Springfield, MA, USA
* 809 N. Bethlehem Pike, P.O. Box 857, Springhouse, PA 19477.
E-mail address: bcutilli@yahoo.com

Nurs Clin N Am 55 (2020) 267–282
https://doi.org/10.1016/j.cnur.2020.02.007
0029-6465/20/© 2020 Elsevier Inc. All rights reserved.
nursing.theclinics.com

patient education (verbal, written, games, etc.). The nurse synthesizes the patient's concerns/learning needs, teaching strategies based on the learner's assessment, and evaluation feedback to implement individualized, effective, and efficient education. If this synthesis is successful, verbal patient education resembles a relaxed conversation on a health topic rather than a lecture, and written education is simple, informative, and engaging.

ASSESSMENT—GET TO KNOW YOUR PATIENTS AND CAREGIVERS

The first component in the patient education process is assessment.[1] For nurses to effectively teach, they need to know the patient's and caregiver's concerns and knowledge by consistently assessing during each patient education encounter. However, this component of patient education is often underutilized, leading to patients and caregivers being "talked at" rather than fully engaged during education.[2] Tools used by health care professionals to evaluate patient education material often focus on how the information promotes patient understanding and action.[3] Although meeting the criteria of these tools indicates excellent patient education, the material may not be effective if it does not address the patient's concerns, learned through assessment.

Nurses know the basic aspects of assessment, driven by regulatory requirements and routinely completed on admission:

1. Motivation/desire to learn
2. Religious/cultural beliefs
3. Emotional Barriers
4. Cognitive/physical limitations
5. Communication barriers[4]

However, this basic assessment does not provide enough information to understand the patient's and caregiver's perspectives to plan education to address concerns and build on previous knowledge. One of the most important and first questions to ask patients and caregivers is "What are you worried about?"[5] This demonstrates that the nurse is listening and is focused on the patient's and caregiver's perspective. For the patients undergoing a total knee replacement, this question will provide a "window" into where they are in the educational process. For example, patients may reply that they are concerned about having uncontrolled pain or the care provided to their loved one with Alzheimer will not be sufficient while they are recovering. Once these concerns are addressed, a relationship with the patient develops and the patient becomes more receptive to teaching, which the clinician feels is important.[6]

Engaging Patients Through Assessment

Assessment is an iterative process where patients and caregivers are constantly engaged to obtain their perspectives/knowledge. This information is used as a tool to connect prior knowledge to new knowledge to promote learning.[7] Repeated assessment also provides an opportunity for the nurse to address incorrect current knowledge. For example, a patient, C.C., needed a cortisone injection into the shoulder, but she was very reluctant because she had heard from multiple sources that these injections are very painful. C.C. saw a nurse practitioner (NP) who asked her about her experience with steroid injections. C.C. said she had injections in her knee but heard the shoulder is very painful. NP explained that shoulder injection C.C. would be receiving is not painful and that freezing spray would be used. The NP built on C. C's knowledge by comparing how this injection would be done compared with her knee injections and exactly what C.C. would feel, to correct her perception of a painful experience. C.C. had the injection with no pain (slight pressure) and went on to a second injection weeks later with the same experience. If C.C.'s knowledge had not been assessed, she probably would have not had the injections and her clinical course would be been prolonged and painful.

Application of Assessment Concepts

The assessment of the patient needs to focus on previous experience with the health concern and system. For example, J.D. is having a knee replacement. The nurse guides J.D. through open-ended prompts ("Tell me what you know about knee replacement.") to elicit any experience/knowledge. J.D. shares that his brother had a knee replacement 10 years ago. His brother did well in outpatient therapy with a home exercise plan (raising leg, bending knee); however he had terrible pain (only used pain pills) immediately after surgery. The nurse uses this information to teach J.D. about current ways to management pain with pharmacologic and nonpharmaco-logic interventions (**Box 1**).

The nurse and patient in this example have an effective teaching session in the context of a conversation—the nurse uses the patient's knowledge of knee replace-ment to provide new information.

Health Literacy

The health literacy of patients and caregivers needs to be considered throughout the education process.[8] In Healthy People 2010 health literacy was defined as "the degree to which individuals have the capacity to obtain, process, and understand basic health information and services needed to make appropriate health decisions."[9] According to the National Assessment of Adult Literacy approximately one-third of the population has basic or below basic health literacy.[10] The characteristics associated with lowest health literacy include age greater than 65 years, low income and educational achieve-ment, race (Black, Hispanic, American Indian/Native, and multiracial), did not speak English before formal education, rate their health as poor, use public insurance (ie, Medicare, Medicaid) or no insurance, and seek print and nonprint sources of health information less often.[10]

For the most part, nurses rely on their judgment to determine the health literacy of patients and caregivers; however, this is problematic because research shows that nurses overestimate patients' health literacy.[11] A solution for this problem would be assessing the health literacy of all patients. However, after almost 3 decades of health literacy assessment tool development, there is still no gold standard to use in the clin-ical setting. To address this issue, the concept of Health Literacy Universal Precau-tions was developed.[12] Health Literacy Universal Precautions recommends treating all patients as if they may have difficulty understanding how to manage their health concerns. From a patient education perspective, nurses need to teach all patients as if they have low health literacy.

Motivational Interviewing

Motivational interviewing (MI) is another tool to aid in assessing patients for educa-tional needs. MI is described as a way of communicating with patients to elicit what motivates them to make health behavioral changes.[13] This approach comes from psychology/psychiatry. Although not every aspect of MI is applicable in a fast-paced health care setting, there are 4 pertinent elements identified through the acronym OARS:

Box 1
Patient assessment of pain management knowledge

Nurse: You mentioned that your brother had terrible pain after his knee replacement. Tell me what you know about controlling pain after surgery.

J.D.: I don't want to have the terrible pain like my brother; however, I am afraid that I will get addicted to pain pills. I have heard that it is better to not take pain meds even if I am in terrible pain. I don't know what to do.

Nurse: I can understand your concerns about pain and becoming addicted. There are other ways to control pain that do not involve pain pills...how do you feel about discussing them?

J.D.: I have never heard of other ways. In the past with other surgeries I have had, pain pills are the only thing that worked. Do these other ways work?

Nurse: Yes, we have research that shows there are other ways to help control your pain. I am wondering if you have used some of these in the past when you have had short pain episodes such as muscle cramp or stubbed toe. What do you do when this happens?

J.D.: For a cramp, I move around and take deep breaths. For a stubbed toe, I just stay still for 30 seconds, hold my foot and deep breathe.

Nurse: When you are uncomfortable after the surgery, try changing your position (move around) and take nice slow deep breaths. What else helps you relax or distract yourself?

J.D.: I meditate, listen to music, or watch TV.

Nurse: Pain is usually less when you are relaxed. After surgery try meditation, music, and TV for pain relief. Hopefully, changing position, deep breathing, meditation, watching TV, and listening to music will lessen your pain so you can take less pain pills. You want to be able to move around and do therapy right after surgery.

J.D.: What if the pain is too bad?

Nurse: Ice or heat can also help decrease pain. Ice can be used anywhere on your body that helps. Heat can be used anywhere except near or on the incision. Although I know you want to avoid pain pills, you may need to take a bit more if your pain is keeping you from moving around and doing therapy.

J.D.: Ok, ice has helped me in the past. I will think about using more pain pills if I need to.

Nurse: We have talked about several ways to control pain after your knee replacement. Tell me what you think will work for you.

J.D.: To help lessen my pain, I can move around/change my position, take deep breaths, meditate, use ice or heat, and distract myself with music or TV.

Nurse: Sounds like you have a plan for ways to control your pain in addition to pain pills.

O-pen-ended question—encourages sharing of information
A-ffirmation—provides positive feedback to support patient
R-eflection—demonstrates listening by clinician
S-ummary—synthesizes and confirms ideas shared by patient

The OARS approach engages patients/families to aid in identifying motivations for health behaviors.[13] OARS is demonstrated in **Box 2**.

ASSESSING FOR APPROPRIATE TEACHING STRATEGIES/METHODS

Besides assessing for patient education content, it is important to understand the teaching strategies/methods desired by the target audience.[1] Although patient preferences for learning health information are often asked when patient have the initial health care encounter, this should not be considered a completed assessment. The

---

Box 2
Assessment example of motivational interviewing

S.N. was due in the osteoporosis clinic a year ago for follow-up. She makes an appointment because she is having pain in her hip.

Nurse: Hi S.N.! My name is Joe Smith and I am the nurse who will be working with you today. I am so glad that you came in. (affirmation) Tell me what brings you in today? (open-ended question)

S.N.: I have hip pain. It started a couple months ago and has gotten worse. It keeps me up at night.

Nurse: (Nodding his head while S.N. talks) Do you do anything that makes the pain better? (open-ended question)

S.N.: I take ibuprofen, move around, and try to distract myself with music or TV.

Nurse: So, your hip pain started a couple months ago and has steadily worsened and now keeps you awake at night. Ibuprofen, moving around, and distraction helps you manage the pain. (Summary) Do you want to tell me anything else?

S.N.: I am very upset about my hip. It hurts so bad at night; I start to cry.

Nurse: It sounds like this is very painful for you. (reflection) Let's start talking about the cause of the pain and how to control the pain.

---

patients/caregivers should be assessed for preferred learning method for each teaching session if choices of methods are available. The patients'/caregivers' preference may change based on the knowledge and skill to be learned. For learning about medications, patients and caregivers may prefer reading or listening. For a dressing change, the patients/caregivers may prefer demonstration. Research is demonstrating that a multimodal approach to educating patients is more effective than a single mode such as verbal or written.[14,15]

Specific Assessment for NAON Patient Education Manuals

Assessment is a critical component in the development of written materials for a specific patient population. The National Association of Orthopedic Nurses (NAON) revised the patient education manuals for knee, hip, and shoulder replacements (total knee replacement, total hip replacement, and total shoulder replacement) and spine surgery in 2018. During the revision process, the NAON Education Project Team asked patients about the information they wanted in the manuals. They scripted the dialogue to use when asking patients for the manuals' content (**Box 3**).

Patients recommended content that focused on what the patient could do to prepare for surgery (diet, exercise, home preparation) and recovery at home. The patients

---

Box 3
Script to assess manual content

Hello, [Introduce yourself if you don't already have a relationship with the patient]. My name is (insert name), and I'm the (insert job title). I'm a member of the National Association of Orthopedic Nurses and one of our projects is to enhance our patient education materials on orthopedic surgeries. I'd like to gather information from you about what you think is important to learn about your surgery before, during and after it. This is not a formal survey. Your comments will only be shared with the small group that is working on patient education. Your comments will help our patient education group develop materials that patients can easily understand about their surgery. Do you mind if I ask you a few questions?

reviewed other content areas of the manuals (ie, surgery description, medical evalua-tion, incision care, pain and constipation management) and provided feedback. This assessment provided the foundation for the patient behaviors and content that would be used in the next phases of revising the manuals: planning and implementation.

PLANNING/IMPLEMENTATION

The next 2 components of the patient education process are planning and implemen-tation.[1] Nurses are most comfortable and familiar with the implementation component of patient education—teaching a topic. However, successful implementation depends on effective planning. Nurses use the assessment from patients/caregivers to develop patient-centered/individualized teaching plans based on mutually determined goals.[1] The goals are specific patient behaviors that result from the education, chosen before the educational content, and strategies are determined.

Patient Behaviors

Identifying specific patient behaviors for patient education may not be intuitive for nurses. In addition, nurses may not think of patient education from this perspective. However, effective education can be only be developed once the desired behaviors are identified. One can use the analogy of planning a vacation to gain greater under-standing of the planning component of patient education. When planning a vacation, the navigation for the trip cannot be determined until the final destination of the trip is set. When planning patient education, the teaching plan (navigation) cannot be com-plete until the patient behaviors (final destination) are identified. Thus, well-defined pa-tient behaviors are essential for evidence-based patient and family education.

For example, a young male patient, W.H., is having surgery for a fractured wrist. He is Spanish speaking, has had a brain injury and wrist surgery, and has a caregiver (his wife who speaks English). From the initial assessment, the nurse begins to develop pa-tient behaviors (with patient/caregiver) and individualized teaching plan:

- Mutually determined patient behaviors examples
  - Complete pre-op medical evaluation
  - Use wrist splint to protect from further injury and lessen pain
  - Use pharmacologic and nonpharmacologic pain management techniques
- Teaching plan examples
  - Spanish interpretation/translation services
  - Caregiver involvement, repetition, and short teaching sessions
  - Surgery information designed with prior knowledge incorporated
  - Effective teaching strategies
    - Verbal
    - Written

The nurse will refine the patient behaviors and teaching plan as she continually as-sesses during each educational topic.

NAON Patient Education Manuals: Patient Behaviors

For the revision of the NAON patient education manuals, the NAON Education Project Team worked with patients to determine patient behaviors and corresponding con-tent. Through this process, they realized that the desired behaviors were similar for to-tal joint replacements and spine surgeries. Thus, the NAON Education Project Team developed a common group of patient behaviors to be used in each manual (total knee replacement, total hip replacement, total shoulder replacement, and spine surgery). Developing the behaviors was a challenging and thought-provoking activity. **Boxes 4–6** provide examples of mutually determined patient behaviors for the 4 NAON patient education manuals.

Content and Teaching Methods

The patient behaviors and learning needs drive the content development and teaching methods. Current patient education research demonstrates that individualized/ patient-centered content and multimodal delivery methods are effective teaching strategies.[14–17] The previous patient example provides an opportunity to show how current research is translated into practice. W.H.'s educational content is individualized, interpreted into Spanish, and communicated in a simple repetitive manner. His wife's education about his care is communicated in English. Both W.H. and his wife receive written information (Spanish and English) to support the verbal patient education. This is an example of a multimodal (written and verbal), patient-centered approach to patient education.

Health Literacy Universal Precautions

The concept of Health Literacy Universal Precautions is a very important consideration for the planning/implementation stages of the patient education process. This concept is part of the Health Literacy Universal Precautions Toolkit from the Agency for Healthcare Research and Quality (AHRQ).[12] The precautions recommend that nurses teach all patients as if they have low health literacy and use specific strategies to meet health literacy demands of the target audience.

Using Marketing Concepts in Patient Education

The goal of learning is a change in behavior (knowledge, skills, attitudes) that occurs as a result of exposure to stimuli.[1] Marketing works toward the same goal—changing behavior that results in the purchase/use of a product or service.[18] Nursing may find more effective ways to educate patients by looking at the field of marketing.

Box 4
Preoperative behaviors

Preoperative behaviors
- Complete medical evaluation and medical testing per provider instructions
- Schedule outpatient physical therapy and other follow-up appointments
- Arrange transportation to appointments (therapy, health care providers)
- Arrange for support system to provide care at home
- Obtain sufficient routine medications for recovery period
- Arrange for durable medical equipment
- Prepare home for mobility with medical equipment
- Complete exercises as instructed
- Develop plan to manage pain before, during, and after with health care team (pharmacologic and nonpharmcologic modalities)
- Develop plan with health care team to avoid medications that may lead to complications
- Describe healthy lifestyle behaviors with health care team to promote healing (smoking cessation, wright management)
- Prepare skin for surgery as instructed by provider
- Describe ways they can minimize infections (hand hygiene, wound care, and pets)
- State signs and symptoms of blood clots and clots prevention
- Describe expected activity level (dangle, stand, sit in chair, walk) following surgery
- Describe anesthesia options
- Describe multimodal ways to minimize and treat constipation

---

Box 5
During hospitalization behaviors

- Use multimodal pain management to obtain rest and participate in therapy
- Maintain adequate nutrition to promote healing
- Exercise as instructed
- Use assistive devices (walker, cane)
- Complete bed exercises (isometric, deep breathing)
- Get out of bed day of surgery
- Teach back/demonstrate complications prevention (incisional infection, DVT, uncontrolled pain, constipation)
- Teach back/demonstrate all self-care strategies to be used at home (mobility, pain management, wound care)
- State medicines' uses, side effects, and possible allergic reaction
- Describe when to call the surgeon and 911
- Demonstrate strategies to minimize swelling

Beckwith in his book, "Selling the Invisible," states that the key to success in the service industry is to build relationships.[18] Health care is a service industry, and success in having health information change health behavior depends on relationships built with patients.

Heath and Heath highlight in their book, "Made to Stick," ideas that survive over time.[19] These ideas have the following characteristics:

Box 6
Caring for self at home

- Attend outpatient physical therapy and other follow-up appointments
- Use and adjust transportation to appointments (therapy, health care providers) as needed
- Use and adjust support system as needed
- Demonstrate safe use of durable medical equipment
- Complete exercises as instructed
- Implement plan to manage pain (pharmacologic and nonpharmacologic modalities)
- Implement healthy lifestyle behaviors to promote healing (smoking cessation, weight management)
- Demonstrate strategies to minimize infections (hand hygiene, wound care, and pets)
- Demonstrate clot prevention and call provider if clots are suspected.
- Demonstrate increased activity daily
- Demonstrate multimodal ways to minimize and treat constipation
- Report medicines' adverse and allergic reaction
- Demonstrate when to call the surgeon and 911, if needed
- Demonstrate ways to minimize swelling
- Demonstrate incision care

- Simple basic message
- Unexpected aspect
- Concrete clear ideas
- Credible
- Emotional
- Story

Health care needs to design patient education with these characteristics to make education "stick" over time. Godin also emphasizes the importance of telling a story and recommends stating your health message so it fits into your patient's world view.[20] Godin's recommendation requires nurses to get to know their patients so health information can be placed in the context of the patient's world. The example in **Box 7** demonstrates the use of these marketing techniques in patient education. The nurse builds a relationship with the patient; teaches from the patient's world view; and uses a simple message, concrete ideas, emotion, and a story.

Verbal Education

Multiple resources recommend using specific verbal communication strategies for all patients/caregivers, especially those with low health literacy. Most of the strategies listed here are part of the plain language approach and focus on verbal education.[8,12,21]

- Use language familiar to patients/caregivers
- Avoid medical terminology

Box 7
Marketing techniques used in patient education

Nurse Bill: How are you today Mr Jones?

Mr Jones: I am good, Bill. How are you?

Nurse Bill: Good. What did you think of the ball game last night?

Mr Jones: Great game! Glad they won.

Nurse Bill: Agree. Fun game to watch. Yesterday we discussed how you did pin care with your nephew a few years. Are you ready to continue pin care teaching today?

Mr Jones: Yes, I am.

Nurse Bill: Good, let's get started. I like to think pin care is like a baseball game, specifically running the bases. I was watching the game last night when Roberts was running the bases. Did you see when he gave the crazy handshake coming into the dugout...it was hilarious. (laughing)

Mr Jones: It was very funny (laughing).

Nurse Bill: When he was going around the bases, he would get enough of a lead to make it to the next base but not too far that he couldn't make it back to the prior base when he was stealing or advancing on a hit. He would work his way around the bases avoiding being tagged out. Pin care is very similar. When you do pin care, you want to clean enough to gently remove crusting but not too much that you make open areas for bacteria to enter. The key is to clean gently. Does that make sense?

Mr Jones: Yeah, I get the idea...clean gently.

Nurse Bill: Let me show you pictures of a pin site prior to being cleaned and after cleaning. See how the crusts are removed but there are no new open areas for bacteria to get in.

Mr Jones: Yes, I see how this is done. It is similar to running the bases during a baseball game.

- Teach most important information first
- Make teaching as simple as possible without losing meaning
- Teach only "need to know" versus "nice to know" information
- Organize content logically
- Chunk information into short sections
- Use short words and sentences
- Use conversational tone
- Introduce each topic
- Use visuals to enhance teaching
- Leave "pauses' in the conversation for the patient to reflect/think of questions

Written Education

Although similar strategies are used for written materials, there are additional criteria for evidence-based written and audiovisual (AV) patient education materials. AHRQ has developed a tool, PEMAT, which lists evidence-based criteria for written and AV materials.[3] The tool is unique because it breaks the criteria into 2 different components: understandability and actionability. The tool for written materials is located in **Table 1**. The tool and instructions for written and AV can be found at the following URL: https://www.ahrq.gov/professionals/prevention-chronic-care/improve/self-mgmt/pemat/pemat-p.html.

Another tool for evaluating patient education materials is called the Suitability Assessment of Materials (SAM).[22] In addition to the PEMAT criteria, the SAM assesses literacy demand, learning stimulation, and cultural appropriateness. Literacy demand refers to the reading level of written material. This is the area that has changed since the development of the SAM. Rather than prescribing a certain reading level for excellent patient education, the current approach is to make the reading level and reading ease as low as possible without losing meaning.[8] The reading level refers to a specific grade level, and the reading ease provides a number for overall how easy the material is read (good score is 70–100). Because recognizing reading levels and reading ease is not a common practice in nursing, when developing written materials, the nurse should use a tool to determine the approximate reading level. Patient education experts often use the Simple Measure of Gobbledygook (https://www.online-utility.org/english/readability_test_and_improve.jsp),[23] Dale-Chall Readability Formula (http://www.readabilityformulas.com/free-dale-chall-test.php),[24] or Fry Graph Readability Formula (http://www.readabilityformulas.com/free-fry-graph-test.php).[25]

Learning simulation focuses on engaging the patient. This can be done by promoting interaction (test knowledge, problem solve), modeling behavior, and having tasks or behaviors patients can do (broken into steps). Material that is culturally appropriate matches the culture of the audience, shows appropriate cultural images and examples, and is suitable for the target population (socioeconomically and culturally). The SAM tool and instructions can be found in the text by Doak, Doak, and Root.[22]

NAON Patient Education Manual Content

NAON revised the patient education manuals using the assessment information and a synthesis of the tools and other evidence-based strategies. The NAON Education Project Team wrote content that promoted the achievement of specific patient behaviors. **Box 8** presents the specific patient behavior and corresponding content for pain management. The reading level for a section on pain management went from 11th grade in the original manual to 7th in the revised, and the reading ease went from 52 to 85. In addition, the presentation of information was changed to place the

Table 1
Patient Education Assessment of Materials Tool

	Understandability		
Item #	**Item**	**Response Options**	**Rating**
Topic: Content			
1	The material makes its purpose completely evident.	Disagree = 0, Agree = 1	
2	The material does not include information or content that distracts from its purpose.	Disagree = 0, Agree = 1	
Topic: Word Choice & Style			
3	The material uses common, everyday language.	Disagree = 0, Agree = 1	
4	Medical terms are used only to familiarize audience with the terms. When used, medical terms are defined.	Disagree = 0, Agree = 1	
5	The material uses the active voice.	Disagree = 0, Agree = 1	
Topic: Use of Numbers			
6	Numbers appearing in the material are clear and easy to understand.	Disagree = 0, Agree = 1, No numbers = N/A	
7	The material does not expect the user to perform calculations.	Disagree = 0, Agree = 1	
Topic: Organization			
8	The material breaks or "chunks" information into short sections.	Disagree = 0, Agree = 1, Very short material[a] = N/A	
9	The material's sections have informative headers.	Disagree = 0, Agree = 1, Very short material[a] = N/A	
10	The material presents information in a logical sequence.	Disagree = 0, Agree = 1	
11	The material provides a summary.	Disagree = 0, Agree = 1, Very short material[a] = N/A	
Topic: Layout & Design			
12	The material uses visual cues (eg, arrows, boxes, bullets, bold, larger font, highlighting) to draw attention to key points.	Disagree = 0, Agree = 1, Video = N/A	
Topic: Use of Visual Aids			
15	The material uses visual aids whenever they could make content more easily understood (eg, illustration of healthy portion size).	Disagree = 0, Agree = 1	
16	The material's visual aids reinforce rather than distract from the content.	Disagree = 0, Agree = 1, No visual aids = N/A	
17	The material's visual aids have clear titles or captions.	Disagree = 0, Agree = 1, No visual aids = N/A	

(continued on next page)

Table 1
(continued)

Understandability

Item #	Item	Response Options	Rating
18	The material uses illustrations and photographs that are clear and uncluttered.	Disagree = 0, Agree = 1, No visual aids = N/A	
19	The material uses simple tables with short and clear row and column headings.	Disagree = 0, Agree = 1, No tables = N/A	

Total Points: _____.
Total Possible Points: _____.
Understandability Score (%): _____ (Total Points/Total Possible Points x 100).

Actionability

Item #	Item	Response Options	Rating
20	The material clearly identifies at least one action the user can take.	Disagree = 0, Agree = 1	
21	The material addresses the user directly when describing actions.	Disagree = 0, Agree = 1	
22	The material breaks down any action into manageable, explicit steps.	Disagree = 0, Agree = 1	
23	The material provides a tangible tool (eg, menu planners, checklists) whenever it could help the user take action.	Disagree = 0, Agree = 1	
24	The material provides simple instructions or examples of how to perform calculations.	Disagree = 0, Agree = 1, No calculations = NA	
25	The material explains how to use the charts, graphs, tables, or diagrams to take actions.	Disagree = 0, Agree = 1, No charts, graphs, tables, or diagrams = N/A	
26	The material uses visual aids whenever they could make it easier to act on the instructions.	Disagree = 0, Agree = 1	

Total Points: _____.
Total Possible Points: _____.
Actionability Score (%): _____ (Total Points/Total Possible Points x 100).

[a] A very short print material is defined as a material with two or fewer paragraphs and no more than 1 page in length.
From PEMAT for Printable Materials (PEMAT-P). Content last reviewed October 2013. Agency for Healthcare Research and Quality, Rockville, MD.http://www.ahrq.gov/professionals/prevention-chronic-care/improve/self-mgmt/pemat/pemat-p.html.

most important information first and formatting moved from paragraphs to bullet points. Patient feedback on the manual was obtained throughout the revision process to assure that it met the needs of the target audience. The manuals are on the NAON Website and can be found at the following URL: http://www.orthonurse.org/page/patient-education.

Box 8
Patient behavior: implement plan to manage pain (pharmacologic and nonpharmacologic modalities) National Association of Orthopedic Nurses, Patient Education Manual, Postoperative Spine

Pain Management
  What can I do to lessen the pain?
  There are many ways to lessen pain. Below is a list of options. Work with the health care team to find the best ways.
  • Ice
    ○ Ice is a good way to lessen pain.
    ○ Ice should be used right after surgery around the incision.
    ○ Ice should never be placed directly on bare skin. Keep ice packs wrapped in a towel or placed over clothing.
    ○ Ice should be continued as long as you have pain from surgery.
    ○ Ice for 20 minutes at a time. Ice should be off at least 20 minutes.
  • Stay active
    ○ Get up and move around as instructed.
    ○ Change positions to help reduce pain.
  • Relaxation
    ○ Rest—make sure you are getting enough, good quality sleep.
    ○ Breathing exercises—slow, deep breathing can reduce stress and pain.
    ○ Guided imagery—a method to guide your mind and help you relax.
    ○ Meditation—this can help focus your mind and let you relax.
    ○ Music—find music that is calming or enjoyable to you. This can also help with relaxation.
  • Pills
    ○ Narcotic pain medicine (opioids).
      ■ Use right after surgery.
      ■ Stop using as soon as possible after surgery.
    ○ Nonsteroidal antiinflammatory drugs (NSAIDs)
      ■ The most common are ibuprofen (Advil) and naproxen (Aleve).
      ■ Talk with your doctor if you have a history of kidney problems, bleeding problems, or NSAID allergy.
      ■ Choose either ibuprofen or naproxen. Do not take both at the same time.
    ○ NSAIDs can be taken with narcotics. NSAIDs can help decrease use of narcotics (opioids).
      ■ Acetaminophen (Tylenol) controls pain differently from narcotics and NSAIDs.
        • Talk with your doctor about taking acetaminophen if you have a history of liver problems or acetaminophen allergy.
        • Acetaminophen can be taken with narcotics and NSAIDs. It can help decrease narcotic used (opioids).
        • Some opioids contain acetaminophen (Percocet, Norco, etc.). Be sure to count any acetaminophen in your narcotics toward your daily dose limit.

Data from National Association of Orthpaedic Nurses. Patient Education Manual: Postoperative Spine. 2018. Available at: file:///Users/cutillic/Downloads/PostoperativeSpine_Manual_NAON1118%20(3).pdf. Accessed June 2, 2019.

EVALUATION

The final component of the patient education process is evaluation. Unfortunately, this phase is often overlooked or executed by simply asking patients/caregivers if they understand. This is a missed opportunity to determine a patient's knowledge of self-care and disease management. Various methods of evaluation can be integrated into the education process: knowledge tests, demonstration, and teach back.[2] The teach back technique is one of the most recommended methods to verify patient understanding.

There is an "art" to implementing teach back. The Website "Always Use Teach-Back! Training Toolkit" (https://www.teachbacktraining.org/) provides basic information and training modules.[26] However, the nurse can use some of the nuances of the technique to enhance teach back. First, teach back should be done in a manner so that the patient does not feel like they are being tested. Second, teach back should address knowledge, attitude, and behavior.[27] Third, the nurse needs to take responsibility if a patient does not understand and adjust the teaching until the patient/caregiver does understand.

There are various ways to respectfully prompt patients to share knowledge during teach back. These strategies focus on the reason for the teach back, the nurse's ability to teach, effectiveness of teaching tools, amount of information, or sharing with caregivers. Here are examples of teach back prompts that do not make the patient feel like they are being tested:

- I want to make sure that I have been clear in my teaching, can you tell me how to clean your pin sites?
- We are using a new booklet to help teach you about spine surgery, I want to make sure the booklet works. Can you tell me 3 things you must do to help your recovery from surgery?
- We have covered lots of information about your hip replacement...I would be overwhelmed. I am wondering if you can you tell me 3 things you need to do before surgery?
- Your son will be coming in this afternoon, tell me what you will tell him about your arm exercises after your shoulder replacement.

Teach back should be thought of as a process where patients'/caregivers' knowledge, attitude, and behavior are addressed.[27] For example, patients going home with incision care will tell the nurse that they clean the incision with mild soap and water to prevent infection. When describing exactly how to clean the incision, patients may state that they need to scrub the incision. Because the nurse had the patients teach back exactly how to clean the incision (behavior), the nurse can reteach incorrect information such as "scrubbing" the incision.

The final step in the "art" of teach back is taking responsibility for teaching. If a patient does not understand, the nurse must use various teaching methods until the patient does understand. If the patient cannot understand, then the nurse is responsible to communicate this information to the health care team so that care can be provided by others (caregivers or facility).

The following video emphasizes the importance of teach back and the difference it can make in clinical outcomes: https://vimeo.com/48471644.[28]

SUMMARY

Patient education is a process (assessment, planning, implementation, and evaluation) in which each component is necessary.[1] Nursing has a tendency to focus most efforts on implementation, less on assessment, planning, and evaluation. Feedback from nurses in the postacute setting consistently highlights the ineffectiveness of the current approach to patient education, reporting that patients do not know how to care for themselves. It is time to fully use all components of the patient education process to support knowledge and skill acquisition for self-care.

Approaching patient education as an "art" and "science" provides the foundation for effective teaching. The "art" focuses on the nuances of engaging patients and continually assessing the knowledge/skills/experience/preferred learning methods with health concerns (arthritis, joint surgery, fractures, etc.). The "art" is also involved in determining "need to know" versus "nice to know" health information, incorporating marketing concepts (eg, building relationships, storytelling, simple basic message, patients' world views, emotion), and completing teach back without the patient feeling tested.[8,18–20,26]

The "science" of patient education incorporates evidence-based strategies into the components of the patient education process. The PEMAT and SAM as well as recent research studies provide evidence for the planning, implementation, and evaluation aspects of the process.[3,22] Nurses need to implement patient education that has plain language (common everyday words, nonmedical jargon) and short words and sentences, describes patient actions, and is patient centered and multimodal.[14–17,21] Evidence shows that teach back and demonstration are effective evaluation strategies.[2] The key to educating patients effectively is using "art" and "science" to create and teach health information using the patient education process: assessment, planning, implementation, and evaluation.

DISCLOSURE

The author has nothing to disclose.

REFERENCES

1. Bastable SB, Gonzales KM. Overview of education in health care. In: Bastable SB, editor. Essentials of patient education. 2nd edition. Burlington (MA): Jones & Bartlett Learning; 2017. p. 10–2.
2. London F. No Time to teach: the essence of patient and family education for health care providers. 2nd edition. Atlantic (GA): Pritchett & Hull Associates, Inc.; 2016. p. 15–164.
3. Agency for Healthcare Research and Quality (AHRQ). Patient Education Material Assessment Tool (PEMAT) 2015. Rockville (MD). Available at: https://www.ahrq.gov/professionals/prevention-chronic-care/improve/self-mgmt/pemat/pemat-p.html. Accessed June 2, 2019.
4. The Joint Commission. Joint Commission standards: hospital chapter provision of care 2019. Oakbrook Terrace (IL): PC02.03.01.
5. Ronan B. Will they actually use it? Teaching effectively to ensure action on patient education. J ConsumHealthInternet 2017;21(3):251–62.
6. Rollnick S, Miller WR, Butler CC. Listening. In: Motivational interviewing in health care: helping patient change behavior. New York: Guilford Press; 2008. p. 65.
7. Palis AG, Quiros PA. Adult learning principles and presentation pearls. Middle East Afr J Ophthalmol 2014;21(2):114–22.
8. Parnell TA. Health literacy in nursing: providing person-centered care. New York: Springer Publishing Company, LLC; 2016. p. 115–80.
9. Ratzen SC, Parker RM. Introduction. In: Selden CR, Zorn M, Ratzen SC, et al, editors. National library of medicine current bibliographies in medicine: health literacy. NLMPub. No. CBM 2000-1. Bethesda (MD): National Institutes of Health, U.S. Department of Health and Human Services; 2000.
10. Kutner M, Greenberg E, Jin Y, et al. The health literacy of America's adults: results from the 2003 National assessment of adult literacy 2006. Available at: http://nces.ed.gov/pubsearch/pubsinfo.asp?pubid=2006483. Accessed June 2, 2019.
11. Dickens C, Lambert BL, Cromwell T, et al. Nurse overestimation of patients' health literacy. J HealthCommun 2013;18(suppl1):62–9.
12. Agency for Healthcare Research and Quality (AHRQ). Health literacy universal precautions toolkit. 2nd edition 2015. Rockville (MD). Available at: https://www.ahrq.gov/professionals/quality-patient-safety/quality-resources/tools/literacy-toolkit/index.html. Accessed June 2, 2019.

13. Oregon Health Authority. The OARS model essential communication skills. Center for Health Training; 2010. Available at: http://public.health.oregon.gov/Healthy PeopleFamilies/ReproductiveSexualHealth/Documents/edmat/OARSEssential CommunicationTechniques.pdf. Accessed June 2, 2019.

14. Srisuk N, Cameron J, Ski C, et al. Randomized controlled trial of family-based education for patients with heart failure and their carers. J AdvNurs 2017;73(4): 857–70.

15. Tang TS, Funnell MM, Brown M. Self-management support in "real-world" settings: an empowerment-based intervention. PatientEducCouns 2010;79:178–84.

16. Knier S, Stichler J, Ferber L, et al. Patients' perceptions of the quality of discharge teaching and readiness for discharge. RehabilNurs 2015;40:30–9.

17. Rushton M, Howarth M, Grant MJ, et al. Person-centered discharge instruction following coronary artery bypass graft: a critical review. J ClinNurs 2017;26(5): S206–15.

18. Beckwith H. Selling the invisible: a field guide to modern marketing. New York: Grand Central Publishing; 2012. p. 215–30.

19. Heath C, Health D. Made to stick: why some ideas survive and others die. New York: Random House.; 2008. p. 238–52.

20. Godin S. All marketers are liars (tell stories). New York: Portfolio/Penguin; 2012. p. 1–21, 38–74.

21. Center for Plain Language. Five steps to plain language. 2019. Available at: https://centerforplainlanguage.org/learning-training/five-steps-plain-language/. Accessed June 2, 2019.

22. Doak CC, Doak LG, Root JH. Assessing suitability of materials. In: Teaching patients with low literacy skills. 2nd edition. Philadelphia: J B Lippincott; 1996. p. 41–60.

23. Simple Measure of Gobbledygook (Smog) online calculator. 2009. Available at: https://www.online-utility.org/english/readability_test_and_improve.jsp. Accessed June 2, 2019.

24. Chall-Dale Readability Formula online calculator. 2019. Available at: http://www.readabilityformulas.com/free-dale-chall-test.php. Accessed June2, 2019.

25. Fry Graph Readability Formula online calculator. 2019. Available at: http://www.readabilityformulas.com/free-fry-graph-test.php. Accessed June 2, 2019.

26. Always use teach back. Available at: https://www.teachbacktraining.org/. Accessed June 2, 2019.

27. Peter D, Robinson P, Jordan K, et al. Reducing readmissions using teach-back: enhancing patient and family education. J NursAdm 2015;45(1):35–42.

28. Always use teach-back. Video: Why use teach-back? A patient story-inadvertent overdose. 2012. Available at: https://vimeo.com/48471644. Accessed June 2, 2019.

Moving?

Make sure your subscription moves with you!

To notify us of your new address, find your **Clinics Account Number** (located on your mailing label above your name), and contact customer service at:

Email: **journalscustomerservice-usa@elsevier.com**

800-654-2452 (subscribers in the U.S. & Canada)
314-447-8871 (subscribers outside of the U.S. & Canada)

Fax number: **314-447-8029**

Elsevier Health Sciences Division
Subscription Customer Service
3251 Riverport Lane
Maryland Heights, MO 63043

*To ensure uninterrupted delivery of your subscription, please notify us at least 4 weeks in advance of move.